Communications in Medical and Care Compunetics

Volume 3

Series Editor
Lodewijk Bos, International Council on Medical and Care Compunetics,
Utrecht, The Netherlands

For further volumes:
http://www.springer.com/series/8754

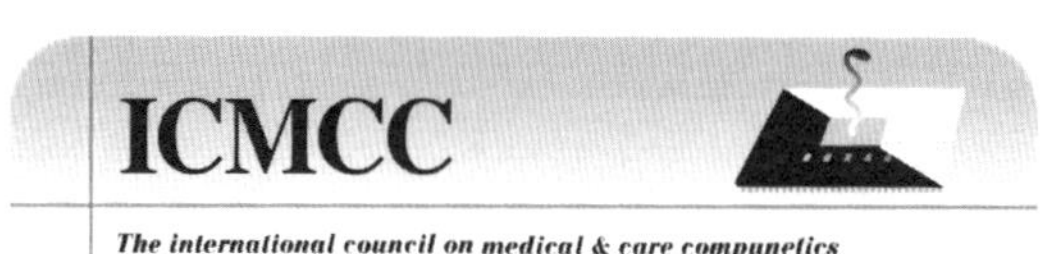

This series is a publication of the International Council on Medical and Care Compunetics.

International Council on Medical and Care Compunetics (ICMCC) is an international foundation operating as the knowledge centre for medical and care compunetics (COMPUting and Networking, its EThICs and Social/societal implications), making information on medicine and care available to patients using compunetics as well as distributing information on the use of compunetics in medicine and care to patients and professionals.

Lodewijk Bos · Adrie Dumay
Leonard Goldschmidt · Griet Verhenneman
Kanagasingam Yogesan
Editors

Handbook of Digital Homecare

Successes and Failures

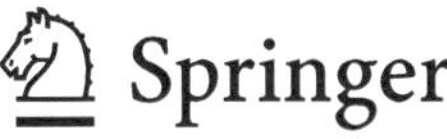 Springer

Lodewijk Bos
International Council on Medical and
  Care Compunetics (ICMCC)
Stationsstraat 38
3511 EG Utrecht
The Netherlands
e-mail: lobos@icmcc.org

Adrie Dumay
TNO/TU Delft
PO Box 5015 Delft
The Netherlands
e-mail: a.c.m.dumaij@tudelft.nl

Leonard Goldschmidt
United States Department of Veterans
  Affairs
Medical Informatics
Health Care System
Miranda Ave. 3801
Palo Alto, CA 94304
USA
e-mail: Leonard.Goldschmidt2@va.gov

Griet Verhenneman
Research Unit Law and Information
  Technology
Sint-Michielsstraat 6, box 3443
3000 Leuven
Belgium
e-mail:
griet.verhenneman@law.kuleuven.be

Kanagasingam Yogesan
Research Director
Australian E-Health Research Centre
2 Verdun Street
Nedlands, WA 6009
Australia
e-mail: Yogi.Kanagasingam@csiro.au

ISSN 2191-3811
ISBN 978-3-642-19646-1
DOI 10.1007/978-3-642-19647-8
Springer Heidelberg Dordrecht London New York

e-ISSN 2191-382X
e-ISBN 978-3-642-19647-8

Library of Congress Control Number: 2011936028

Cover design: eStudio Calamar S.L.

Printed on acid-free paper

Springer is part of Springer Science+Business Media (www.springer.com)

Contents

A High Road to Dutch Healthcare Reform

A. C. M. Dumaij, R. Mooij and J. L. T. Blank

Abstract This study aims to assess the adoption potential of healthcare innovations in their infancy. Such an assessment is useful, since the context of the innovations change rapidly as a result of the health care reform process. Successful innovations comply to a complex system of social, technical, and financial attributes. First we narrow down the vast amount of innovations in healthcare into a review set of innovations and select attributes of successful innovations from literature. Next the compliance of the review set with the attributes is assessed by an expert panel. There exists no metric to objectively measure compliance and empirical data analysis cannot be performed because there are no data. Six innovations with high expectations were assessed: smart homes, eHealth, electronic health records, self management, robotic assisted devices and online health companion contacts. None complied convincingly to all attributes. Innovation in healthcare appears as a multi-level, multi-sector, multi-disciplinary transition and needs both successes and failures to make progress.

Keywords Healthcare · Innovation · Adoption · Reform

1 Introduction

"The flying Dutchman reigns European healthcare as the inequity gap grows". The most remarkable outcome of the Euro Health Consumer Index 2009 report [1] is no

A. C. M. Dumaij (✉) · J. L. T. Blank
Innovation and Public Sector Efficiency (IPSE) Studies,
Delft University of Technology, Delft, The Netherlands
e-mail: a.c.m.dumaij@tudelft.nl

A. C. M. Dumaij · R. Mooij
TNO, Delft, The Netherlands

Commun Med Care Compunetics (2011) 3: 1–14
DOI: 10.1007/8754_2011_19
© Springer-Verlag Berlin Heidelberg 2011
Published Online: 30 April 2011

doubt the outstanding position of Dutch healthcare, indicating that the ongoing healthcare reform now pays off. The reform creates a strategic role for the health consumer and as such it creates a new model for healthcare delivery. The hypothesis is that the costs of this new model are lower than the costs of supply-driven healthcare, with similar quality of care. The Netherlands started to work on this patient empowerment model early, which now clearly pays off in many areas. However, the Euro Health Consumer Index also shows that there is no evidence to support the cost-reducing hypothesis. Actually, the Netherlands has risen in health-care expenditure to the highest per capita spend in Europe. The expenditure increased in the period 1972–2003 0.5% faster than other economies and the price grew 1.2% more than the price of gross domestic product (GDP). Growth that will increase to approximately 15% of GDP in 2040 under the present healthcare policy [2].

One of the most challenging trends in today's Dutch society is the increasing incidence and prevalence of chronic health conditions. Expected increases in prevalence of 40% in 2025 based on the medium variant population projection compared to 2003 are no exception [3]. The increases are mainly a result of the ageing population: more people get older and people live longer. Parallel to this trend is a relative decrease of employees available to work in healthcare: there are (relatively) less young people. Healthcare provides 13% of Dutch employment, not taking into account jobs in supply industries (pharmaceutics and medical tech-nology). The number of full time equivalent (FTE) jobs increases at an annual rate of over 3%, implying that in 2020 480.000 extra FTEs are needed compared to the 2010 level of about 1.000.000 FTEs [4]. Satisfaction from working in healthcare is very much under pressure as a result of increasing bureaucracy and work load. The result is obvious: prevention of disease is necessary and integrated prevention and care has to be delivered in a more—economical—efficient way, making optimal use of the self management potential of patients.

As of 2004, the Dutch government has spent hundreds of millions of Euro on research and development programmes to improve quality, safety, accessibility and cost containment in both the cure and care sector. In addition, health insurance organisations, the medical technology industry, the IT sector, and banking are developing private and public–private initiatives to innovate within the new healthcare framework. Despite the numerous innovation developments in health-care, little attempt has been made to assess the adoption potential of innovations in their infancy. Such an assessment is useful, since the context of the innovations change rapidly as a result of the health care reform process.

1.1 Objective and Outline of this Chapter

This study aims to assess the adoption potential off healthcare innovations in their infancy.

The core of this chapter takes off with an outline of our research method to narrow down the vast amount of innovations in healthcare into a review set of innovations, to select attributes of successful innovations from literature, and to assess compliance of the review set of innovations with the attributes. Next, an overview is presented of the set of innovations including first evaluation results. The assessment results are presented and discussed.

2 Research Methodology

First, a selection of innovation projects for the review is based on the following criteria:

1. The project has started in the Netherlands after the onset of healthcare reform in January 2006;
2. The project has intended impact at organisation (meso) level and as such makes use of technical and social innovations (micro) within the limits of the healthcare system (macro);
3. The study of the project examines the adoption of the innovation taking place in the healthcare-providing organisation;
4. The project aims to positively effect productivity, quality of care, or quality of labor;
5. The study is empirical in nature and demonstrates quantitative analysis.

Keywords to derive at these projects and studies are like (in Dutch translation and synonyms) healthcare, cure, care, chronic disease, improvement project, transition experiment, innovation, acceleration, breakthrough project. Search strings are constructed from these keywords. The search strings are fed into the internet search engine Google with constrained to Dutch websites. Also a structured public database with innovation descriptions is consulted [5].

Secondly, we draw attributes of successful innovations from healthcare innovation literature [6]. These attributes consist of the standard innovation attributes [7] extended with financial [8] and organisational [9] attributes. Compliance of the innovations with the attributes is given on a three-point scale (green: compliant; yellow: undecided; red: non-compliant) by an expert panel. The panel consisted of a total of eight experts from the field of general medicine, geriatrics, diabetics, nursing, human–machine interfacing, psychology, finance and accounting, computer science, and health policy. All experts have at least 12 years of experience with innovation in healthcare. The compliance assessments were performed in a session with all experts present after discussion until consensus is reached. Innovations with many green labels are expected to be adopted more rapidly than other innovations. Since none of these innovations exist for more than 3 years on a reasonable scale, no empirical analysis can be performed. The list of attributes is shown in Table 1.

Table 1 Innovation attributes with factors that influence success and failure of diffusion [6]

Attribute OF INNOVATION	FACTORS FOR SUCCSES AND FAILURE
Relative advantage	User ability to self-reliant use
	Ethics of diffusion
	Clinical relevance
	Degree of user reward
	Convenience to the patient
	Following on demographics and geography
	Societal impact of diffusion
	Urgency of diffusion
Trialability	Effects of diffusion
	Market intelligence
Observability	Participation of the innovator's network
	Promotion and publicity
Compatibility	Willingness of the professional to adapt behaviour
	Fit with conception of the job of the professional
	Unambiguous objective of the innovation
View of opinion leaders	Perceived support of colleagues
	Perceived support of other professionals
	Perceived support of management
	Perceived support of board of directors
	Willingness of the user to adapt behaviour
	Responsibility of the professional over the innovation
	Formal support by opinion leaders within the organisation responsible for diffusion
Public information	Visibility of outcome
	Scientific standards used
	Focussed target group
	Evidence supporting outcome
Homogeneity of groups	Unambiguous requirements of the patient
	Patient support
	Patient satisfaction
	Patient control over healthcare delivery
	Patient usability
	Unambiguous requirements of the professional
	Unambiguous requirements of the social network of the patient
Standards, roles and social networks	Legal framework supporting diffusion
	Comprehension of diffusion procedures
	Presence of similar innovations
Technical fit	Supporting logistic information systems
	Open technical standards
	Standardisation of technology
	Reliability of technology
Adjustability	Degree of adjustability to the patient's situation
Financial fit	Budget for diffusion
	Materials and equipment
	Pay-back of budget for diffusion
	Market stability during diffusion

(continued)

Table 1 (continued)

Attribute OF INNOVATION	FACTORS FOR SUCCSES AND FAILURE
Competition	Time available to the innovators
	Ownership
	Contribution to efficiency in healthcare
Support organisation	Size
	Structure
	Limited staff turnover
	Number of staff
	Limited administrative load
	Involvement of diffusion co-ordinator
	Experience
Co-operation	User involved
	Professionals involved

3 Innovations

3.1 Aging in Place

Aging in place is a widely recognized social trend requiring healthcare and social support to the elderly [10]. Here we find a kaleidoscope of social and technical innovations under the umbrella terms ambient assisted living and smart homes [11]: screen-to-screen consultation (camcare), assistive devices (to navigate through traffic to put on elastic stockings, to prevent decubitus, to stimulate motion, to wash with dry hand, to prevent falling, to comply to medication prescription, to plan healthcare delivery, etc.), home access management, and also means to stimulate self management and patient empowerment, automated time registration of care delivered, nursing home expertise delivered at home and further differentiation of jobs and responsibilities, involvement of informal care providers, and so on. Van den Broek et al. [11] observe the following about:

- Primary stakeholders (the end users); a general reluctance to use technology, unclear evidence of real benefits of ambient assisted living; an inability to use the appropriate technologies;
- Secondary and tertiary stakeholders (the service providers and industries that supply goods); misunderstanding of the requirements and objectives of devices and services; the lack of standards and references for technological design; the partial broadband coverage in geographic areas;
- Quaternary stakeholders (working in economical and legal context of ambient assisted living); diversity of social, welfare and healthcare systems in Europe, lack of visible value chains, lack of standards and certification, funding and reimbursement of services.

The Dutch Healthcare Inspectorate concludes that a care provider cannot be replaced by technology, that a careful risk assessment is essential with respect to technical infrastructure, suitability of the care processes, training and communication of the provider [12]. Also, the inspectorate reports that implementations are rarely evaluated so effects and user experiences cannot be reported.

3.2 eHealth

eHealth is defined as the services that empower the patient to take responsibility in his or her prevention, cure and care of disease or disability by means of information and communication technology. Types of interventions include remote monitoring of chronic heart failure and diabetes, secondary prevention of coronary heart disease, home monitoring of respiratory conditions and online psychological interventions (e.g., drugs and smoking cessation, anxiety disorders). Recent studies of eHealth for the chronic diseases diabetes management (DBM), chronic heart failure (CHF), and chronic obstructive pulmonary disease (COPD) conclude that healthcare expenditure decreases and quality of life improves when used in combination with (electronic) coaching and self management [13–15]. Adoption of eHealth services will be improved when delivered in combination with other online services, like banking, in a public–private business model. The financial structure of healthcare complicates or even obstructs reimbursement of healthcare services. Also, the myriad of technological standards seriously hamper system-to-system interoperability while progress in harmonization of standards is slow [16].

There are a huge number of studies more or less addressing the effects of eHealth. However, there are only a limited number of studies that systematically analyze cost-benefits from empirical studies and also find positive effects on productivity. A systematic review yields that home telemonitoring of respiratory disease results in an early identification of determinants in patient conditions and control of symptoms, positive attitude of patients and receptiveness [17]. Robust study designs are missing and evidence of effects remain preliminary. Remote monitoring of community dwelling patients with CHF has a positive effect on clinical outcomes and secondary prevention [18–20]. Economic data are missing.

3.3 Electronic Healthcare Record

Electronic healthcare record (EHR) is an innovation in the centre of the political arena for over 20 years. The government views the EHR as an instrument to improve efficiency, quality and safety. The healthcare professionals consider it as administrative burden that potentially makes patients more independent of them. The patients are surprised and confused about the slow rate of implementation. Recent pilot implementations at a national scale reveal imperfections that can be fixed from a technical point of view [21]. The Dutch legislator rejected a law for implementing the EHR nationwide, based on potential violation of privacy rights in April 2011.

3.4 Self Management

In healthcare prosumerism is synonymous with an active form of self management, in the literature also referred to as self care [22]. Self management was introduced by Lau who defines it as stimulating the responsibility of the patient with the aim to maximise his or her potential to health and well being [23]. Self management is a new dimension to the concept of patient empowerment in which a patient co-operates with his or her healthcare practitioner to improve health outcomes [24, 25]. It supports the Copernican transition to bring the patient rather than the healthcare provider to the centre of healthcare [26]. The focus being not on applying medical but behavioural interventions. Self management can only be performed when the patient has a sufficient understanding of his or her health conditions [27]. Also, informed decision support or coaching is a critical aspect of self management, regardless of the fact that the support comes from a peer, health companion, practitioner or (medical) device [28–32]. Self management itself is a dynamic process and it affects the utilization of services, patient satisfaction, and health outcomes. Having a valid and reliable measure is important to understanding the effects of self management. However, there is still a lack of a standardized measurement instruments for the empirical assessment of self management in a general patient population. A number of recent initiatives are taking place to develop self management measurement instruments for the general population. E.g., a self management instrument is proposed for the general population covering six domains such as knowledge, access, advocacy, decision making, health status and outcomes, and literacy [33]. Recent studies reveal that most somatic patients choose for self management with support of a health practitioner who is co-operative, empathic and communicative [34]. Operational guidelines for practitioners are available [35] based on motivational interviewing techniques [36].

3.5 Robotic Assistive Devices

Gates predicts an important role for robotics in healthcare due to recent technological developments (faster and cheaper microprocessors, sensors and actuators) and similarities between the development patterns of the computer business 30 years ago and the robotics industry nowadays [37]. Butter et al. extensively investigated contemporary R&D efforts in health and medical robotics and developed a roadmap for the development of robotics in medicine and healthcare [38]. They identified 21 main innovation areas that can be considered key product/ market combinations from which six representative areas can be regarded ripe for further investigation and road mapping. A framework to identify barriers to the development of robotic assistive devices is available [39]. Most constraining economic factor is the lack of risk capital. This limited availability is probably a result of the reserved attitude of financial organisations towards health robotics manufacturers. This attitude is explained by a combination of high initial investment costs and insecurities of getting return on these investments. A possible public intervention to stimulate the development of health robotics is increasing the availability of risk capital. This can be done by stimulating pilot studies to measure the additional value of robotic technology in healthcare, thereby increasing the chance of reimbursement. Although supporting advanced development and commercialisation phases requires high financial capital with uncertain return, the actual production and launch of products increases public awareness of the potential benefits of health robots and can stimulate financial organisations to also get involved in development. Not only financial support is needed. National agreements on key research themes and improved focus are necessary as well. Co-operation agreements on certain research areas among active health technology companies could probably accelerate product development. This can be achieved by stimulating innovation networks and facilitate in bringing partners together.

The most important technological barrier concerns difficulties in technological feasibility. Due to a lack of standards and platforms in health robotics, developers have to begin from scratch when developing an application. This leads to long development times accompanied with high development costs. The most impeding firm capability is a lack of contact with professional end users and patients. A possible public intervention could be the stimulation of innovation networks and to facilitate connecting partners in development.

The most important legal and political barrier is the lack of reimbursement regulations of health robotics. This insecurity contributes to the reserved character of financial organizations to invest in health robotics. Reimbursement problems evolve from a not yet set balance between clinical benefit of health devices on the one hand and cost-effectiveness studies of new health devices on the other. Accurate reflection of the costs of innovative health devices can contribute to develop more accurate estimates of device acquisition costs and to use those estimates to develop new rates. Another remarkable conclusion in this category of barriers is the relative limited influence of difficulties with clinical trials on the product's innovation process. This limited influence is caused by the limited number of unknown factors in health device development compared to clinical development of drugs in the pharmaceutical- or biotech- industry.

Finally, analysis of the user barriers showed that the complexity of integrating robotic products in the existing environment has a significant influence on the product innovation process. Active involvement of and communication with all future users of the robotic devices can prevent most of the implementation problems. It appears crucial to take into account technical, organizational and human factors in the innovation process.

After analysing the influence of the different barriers we can conclude that economic, technological and firm capability barriers have more influence on the product innovation process than the legal, political and user barriers do. Clear policy recommendations might improve the innovation climate in the robotic health device sector, which in general shows great potential. Last but not least, avoid pitfalls in the road from idea to certified product while innovating medical devices [40].

3.6 Online Health Companion Networks

A comprehensive analysis describes the factors that influence online health companion contact use among people with DBM, CHF, asthma/COPD, rheumatic diseases, renal failure or chronic muscle disorders [41]. Respondents of their study are characterized as follows: they are likely to be a woman; aged around 44; married; Dutch; internet users; diagnosed with rheumatic disorders, asthma or COPD and they tend to have lower incomes compared to the general Dutch population. Respondents report privacy concerns and negative stories as barriers for adoption and disadvantages of using online health companion contact. Additionally, concerns regarding the quality of information are perceived as annoying. Benefits mainly concern the possibility to meet people in a similar situation, recognition for their health problems and obtaining information and sharing experiences. The combination with other healthcare services is a determinant for online health companion contact use as well. If decided to use online health companion contact, the selection of a specific website is among others based on technological preferences. Important characteristics of a website include closed access; discussed topics; easy use; type of users and a clear structure. In general, respondents prefer websites facilitated by a forum and organized by patient organizations. Online health companion contact can increase quality of life and self-management according to experiences of the respondents. They perceive to be better informed, better able to accept their disease, better capable to ask questions to medical doctors, better deal with their situation and to receive an increased amount of social support.

4 Results and Discussion

The values given to the attributes of the innovations by the expert panel are shown in Table 2.

Successful innovations should comply to attribute factors, i.e., high relative advantage, trialability, observability, compatibility, supporting view of opinion leaders, observability, homogeneity of groups, building on standards, supporting roles and social networks, technical fit, adjustability, financial fit, competition, strong support organization and co-operation. Although there are no metrics to measure and compare attribute factors, the compliance should be as complete as possible. Critical conditions for successful implementation of innovations are: maintain innovation instruments, active management involvement and commitment, work by method,

Table 2 Expert rating of attributes of innovations in the Netherlands on a 3-point scale (green: positive; yellow: undetermined; red: negative)

ATTRIBUTE OF INNOVATION	SMART HOMES	eHEALTH	EHR	SELF MANAGEMENT	ROBOTIC ASSISTE	ONLINE CONSUMER
Relative advantage						
Trialability						
Observability						
Compatibility						
View of opinion leaders						
Public information						
Homogeneity of groups						
Standards, roles and social networks						
Technical fit						
Adjustability						
Financial fit						
Competition						
Support organisation						
Co-operation						

include the project manager in the management of the organization, be proactive and creative, measure progress in a simple way, encourage informal ambassadors, communicate with images, seek interaction and reflection, consider the project in the context of the organization, keep the materials and appliances in mind, and negotiate.

Many evaluation studies fail due to poor data collection, missing data and poor methodology [42]. This is not surprising, since innovation as a process comes with a rambling and excessive set of objectives, implementation methods, structures, timelines and finance, often claiming the same resources (personnel, clients, technology, finance). Sometimes objectives are even opposing each other. Objectives are rarely framed in a set of institutional instruments. Especially technical and social innovations are seldom thoroughly evaluated on efficiency effects. Implementation methods are usually practical rather than evidence-based. Transitions are rarely managed processes following the "new rules of the game" rather than pushing forward the "old rules of the game". Innovation implementation programmes usually start with smart objectives and end with enthusiasm but poor results [43]. The actors involved in diffusion of innovation are knowledge institutes and experts, branch organizations, occupational groups, patients and clients, administrators, government policy makers. They come in a variety of combinations and levels of commitment to the innovations. It takes great co-ordination effort to define and create win–win objectives and to derive new infrastructure when policies change [44].

Culture is a key characteristic of an organization or sector and has massive influence on success and failure of innovation. It is argued that creating an innovation culture is a dynamic process in which areas of tension and fundamental innovation dilemmas should meet rather than follow a recipe to implement role models and towards success criteria [45]. Four areas of tension and nine innovation dilemmas are described as follows [45]:

- Market versus technology;
- New versus old problem solving approaches;
- Structured evaluation and monitoring of innovation versus go-with-the-flow way of innovation;
- Freedom versus responsibility in the innovation process.

The innovation dilemmas are:

- Identification with present culture versus openness to diversity;
- Incremental versus radical innovation;
- Technology push versus market pull;
- Large versus small;
- Closed versus open innovation;
- Egalitarian versus hierarchical;
- Process directed versus room for creativity and entrepreneurship;
- Individual versus team performance;
- Short term versus long term.

Making the innovation dilemmas explicit does right to the complexity of innovation and provides a basis for choice. It makes obvious that there exists no single best strategy and that organizations and governments should apply trial and error strategies to make best possible choices.

National programmes create awareness for quality and innovation, and yield new ideas and methods to build new capacity to improve quality in both care and cure sector [46, 47]. The programmes aim to increase productivity in the care sector, using collaborative breakthrough methods and campaign methods. They are needed to trigger a new area of systematic improvement with a new body of knowledge, competences and expertise. Lessons are learned about improvement methods (e.g., plan-do-check-act cycles), internal structure, competencies of implementation directors, evaluation methods, and dissemination and assurance methods. Further beneficial impacts are developing acceptance for and some implementation of standardized measuring and improvement instruments. A programme to develop and introduce integrated reimbursement for diabetes care yielded a model for functional funding [46] and a Better Care Academy was established [48]. However, none of the nationally set targets were achieved as a result of over-ambitious goals, underperforming improvement teams, or inadequate timescale as a consequence of annual budgeting. Progress in projects was delayed by problems in identifying best practices and resistance to improving productivity on the part of caregivers. The resistance was fueled by concerns about diminishing quality of care. Also, programmes to improve dementia care had initially no or limited effect on care from both the caregiver and client point of view due to slow start and lack of inclusion of regional co-operations. A rudimentary cost effectiveness analysis yielded an increase of effort by the caregivers for which there is no reimbursement. All innovation projects on mental diseases failed to commit primary healthcare providers, except for the case of anxiety disorders. This is attributed to the fact that there is little co-operation among caregivers and little integration of care processes [46]. Further causes reported to fail implementation are personnel switch, weak competence mix, poor understanding of output and outcome, lack of communication skills and implementation methods, unrealistic assumption that the 20/80 rule (tipping point) applies, and weak security of results.

5 Conclusion

Evaluation of innovations in their infancy is useful since the context of innovation is under reform. Successful innovations comply to a complex system of social, technical, and financial attributes. There exist no metric to objectively measure compliance and empirical data analysis cannot be performed because there are no data. Six innovations with high expectations were assessed: smart homes, eHealth, electronic health records, self management, robotic assisted devices and online health companion contacts. None complied convincingly to all attributes. Innovation in healthcare appears as a multi-level, multi-sector, multi-disciplinary transition and needs both successes and failures to make progress.

References

1. Björnberg A, Garrofé BC, Lindblad S. Euro health consumer index. Brussels: Health Consumer Powerhouse; 2009. ISBN 978–91-977879–1-8.
2. Douven R, Ligthart M, Mannaerts H, Woittiez I. Een scenario voor de zorguitgaven 2008–2011. Den Haag: CPB; 2006. CPB document 121, ISBN 90–5833-278–0. (In Dutch).
3. de Hollander AEM, Hoeymans N, Melse JM, van Oers JAM, Polder JJ. Zorg voor gezondheid. Volksgezondheid Toekomst Verkenning. Bilthoven: RIVM; 2006. RIVM report number: 270061003, ISBN-10: 90-6960-148-6. (In Dutch).
4. De verzorgingsstaat heroverwogen. Over verzorgen, verzekeren, verheffen en verbinden. Den Haag: Wetenschappelijke Raad voor het Regeringsbeleid, WRR report number 76. ISBN 978-90-5356-926-9. (In Dutch).
5. http://www.zorginnovatieplatform.nl. Visited on April 16, 2010. (In Dutch).
6. Oirschot van R, Sooneus E, Bake J, Kroon R. Kennis(in)kaart. Succes- en belemmerings-factoren voor het versnellen van opschaling van innovaties. Den Haag: Alares; 2010. report number 100422 ZIP ES. (In Dutch).
7. Rogers EM. Diffusion of innovations. New York: Free Press; 2003. ISBN 978-0-7432-2209-9.
8. Cain M, Mittman R. Diffusion of innovation in healthcare. Oakland: California Healthcare Foundation; 2002. ISBN 1-929008-97-X.

9. Ottes L. Verspreiding van innovaties: stimulansen en barrières. In: Weten wat we doen. Verspreiding van innovaties in de zorg. Zoetermeer: Raad voor de Volksgezondheid en Zorg; 2005. ISBN 90–5732-1521. (In Dutch).

10. Blanson Henkemans OA, Alpay LL, Dumaij ACM. Aging in place: self-care in smart home environments. In: Al-Qutayri MA, Editors. Smart Home Systems. Olajnica: In-Tech; 2010. p. 105–120.

11. van den Broek G, Cavallo F, Odetti L, Wehrmann C. Ambient assisted living roadmap. Berlin: VDI/VDE-IT AALiance Office; 2009.

12. Toepassing van domotica in de zorg moet zorgvuldiger. Den Haag: Dutch Healthcare Inspectorate. IGZ reference number 09–57, 2009. (In Dutch).

13. Maas A, Mooij R, Bangma M, Rietkerk O, Berkers F, Verhagen P, Blanson Henkemans O, Pathuis W. Bruggen slaan tussen gezondheid, zorg en vrager. Delft/Leiden: TNO; 2009. report number 34999. (In Dutch).

14. Rövekamp AJM, Valentijn P, Mooij R. eHealthNU. First results from literature and interviews. Leiden: TNO; 2010. (In Dutch: eHealthNU. Eerste resultaten op basis van literatuur en interviews).

15. Landewé C, Philippens M, van Oort G. Inventarisatie in de diabeteszorg. Een overzicht van ervaren barriers, mogelijke oplossingsrichtingen en gewenste functionaliteiten. The Hague: KPN; 2010. (In Dutch).

16. Dumaij ACM, Freriks G. Towards developing a coherent healthcare information infrastructure. In: eHealth in Belgium and in the Netherlands, Proceedings of MIC2002, IOS-press Studies in Health Information and Informatics, vol 93, ISBN 0926-9630, (2002) p. 1–7.

17. Jaana M, Pare G, Sicotte C. Home telemonitoring for respiratory conditions: a systematic review. Am J Manag Care. 2009;15(5):313–20.

18. Clark RA, Inglis SC, McAllister FA, Cleland JG, Stewart S. Telemonitoring or structured telephone support programmes for patients with chronic heart failure: systematic review and meta-analysis. BMJ. 2007;334(7600):942.

19. Martinez A, Evers E, Rojo-Alvarez JL, Figal DP, Garcia-Alberola A. A systematic review of the literature on home monitoring for patients with heart failure. J Telemed Telecare. 2006;12(5):234–41.

20. Neubeck L, Redfern J, Fernandez R, Briffa T, Bauman A, Freedman SB. Telehealth interventions for the secondary prevention of coronary heart disease: a systematic review. Eur J Cardiovasc Prev Rehabil. 2009;16(3):281–9.

21. Dumaij ACM, Haaker T. The electronic locum record for general practitioners. Outcome of an evaluation study in the Netherlands. Int J Med Inf. 2010;79(2010):623–36.

22. Dumaij ACM, Blank JLT Healthcare prosumerism. In: Bos L, Carroll D, Kun L, Marsh A, Roa LM (eds.). Communications in Medical and Care Compunetics, Vol.1. A Liber Amicorum in Memory of Swamy Laxninarayan. Springer, ISBN 978-3-642-15050.

23. Lau DH. Patient empowerment: a patient-centred approach to improve care. Hong Kong Med J. 2002;8(5):372–4.

24. Alpay L, Blanson O, Otten W, Rovekamp T, Dumaij ACM. eHealth applications for patient empowerment in the Netherlands: directions for best practices in the Netherlands. J Telemed Telecare. 2010;16(7):787–91.

25. Aujoulat I, Marcolongo R, Bonadiman L, Deccache A. Reconsidering patient empowerment in chronic illness: a critique of models of self-efficacy and bodily control. Soc Sci Med. 2008;66(5):1228–39

26. Lorig K, Holman M. Self-management education: history, definitions, outcomes and mechanisms. Ann Behav Med. 2003;26:1–7.

27. Redman BK. Patient self-management of chronic disease. Sudbury, MA: Jones and Barlett; 2004.

28. Raats CJ, van Veenendaal H, Versluijs MM, Burgers JS. A generic tool for development of decision aids based on clinical practice guidelines. Patient Educ Couns. 2008;73:413–7.

29. Corbin J, Strauss A. Unending work and care: managing chronic illness at home. San Fransisco: Jossey-Bass Publishers; 1988.
30. Ryan RM, Deci EL. Self-determination theory and the facilitation of intrinsic motivation, social development, and well-being. Am Psychol. 2000;55(1):68–78.
31. Leventhal H, Weinman J, Leventhal EA, Phillips LA. Health psychology: the search for pathways between behavior and health. Ann Rev Psychol. 2008;59:477–505.
32. O'Connor AM, Bennett CL, Stacey D, Barry M, Col NF, Eden KB, Entwistle VA, Fiset V, Holmes-Rovner M, Khangura S, Llewellyn-Thomas H, Rovner D. Decision aids for people facing health treatment or screening decisions. Cochrane database of systematic reviews 2009, issue 3. Art. No.: CD001431. doi: 10.1002/14651858.CD001431.pub2.
33. Loukanova S, Bridges JFP. Empowerment in medicine: an analysis of publications trends 1980–2005. Cent Eur Cent J Med. 2008;3(1):105–10.
34. Carmel M, Peterson C, Robinson R, Sturmberg JP. Care for chronic illness in Australian general practice—focus groups of chronic disease self-help groups over 10 years; implications for chronic care systems reforms. Asia Pac Fam Med. 2009;8:1. doi: 10.1186/1447-056X-8-1.
35. Schaefer J, Miller D, Goldstein M, Simmons L. Partnering in self-management support: a toolkit for clinicians. Institute for Healthcare Improvement, Cambridge, MA; 2009 Available at:http://www.improvingchroniccare.org/downloads/partnering_in_selfmanagement_support_ a_toolkit_for_clinicians.doc.
36. Mesters I. Motivational interviewing: hype or hope. Editor. Health Expect. 2009;5:3–6.
37. Gates B. A robot in every home - The leader of the PC revolution predicts that the next hot field will be robotics. Sci Am. 2007;296:44–51.
38. Butter M, et al. Robotics for healthcare. Leiden: TNO Quality of Life; 2008.
39. Dumaij ACM, Boon WPC, v Blijswijk T, Butter M (2011). Identifying barriers in the innovation process of medical robotics. Submitted.
40. Wieringa FP, Poley MJ, Dumaij ACM and Steen AFW van der (2007). Avoiding pitfalls in the road from idea to certified product (and the harsh clinical environment thereafter) when innovating medical devices. Proceedings of the IEEE Benelux EMBS symposium/Belgian day on biomedical engineering.
41. Dumaij ACM, Tijssen E (2011). Online health companion contact among chronically ill in the Netherlands. Health Technol., pp.1–19, doi 10.1007/s12553-011-0003-2.
42. Vos L, Dückers M, Wagner C. Sneller beter, wat kunnen we ervan leren? Tijdschrift over Kwaliteit en Veiligheid in Zorg. 2008;6:10–4. (In Dutch).
43. Beter Sneller. Tien geleerde lessen uit de praktijk. Den Haag: ZonMW; 2008. ISBN 978–90-6910–247-4. (In Dutch).
44. Zwart E. Achter de geraniums. Forse groei dementerenden thuis: wie neemt de regie?. CC Zorgadviseurs: Arnhem; 2008. ISBN 9789079513017. (In Dutch).
45. Prud'homme van Reine PR, Dankbaar B. A crossvergence perspective on creating cultures of innovation: the dynamic interaction between corporate cultures and regional cultures as drivers for convergence and divergence in innovation management. 5th workshop on international strategy and cross-cultural management, Istanbul, Koç University, 28–29 Sept (2007).
46. Øvretveit J, Klazinga N. Meta-evaluation of ten national quality improvement programmes in The Netherlands 2004–2009. The Hague: The Netherlands Organisation for Health Research and Development (ZonMw); 2010.
47. van der Linden B. Grootschalige kwaliteitsverbetering: lessen uit 10 ZonMW programma's. Kwaliteit in zorg. 2010;2:4–8. (In Dutch).
48. Zorg voor Beter Academie. http://www.zorgvoorbeter.nl/aan-de-slag/academie/. Site visited on 3 June 2010. (In Dutch).

The Epilepsy Project in the Republic of Ireland: Lessons for Digital Homecare

Malcolm J. Fisk

Abstract Sometimes overlooked from within the range of long term conditions that are being addressed via telecare (care service provision mediated by telecommunications technologies) are the needs of people with epilepsy. This chapter reports on a telecare project (the Epilepsy Project) in the Republic of Ireland that, through the use of bed epilepsy sensors, supported the needs of people with epilepsy and their carers at home. The service developed in the Project is now mainstreamed but operates on a relatively small scale. Positive conclusions were drawn in a comprehensive evaluation of the Project that explored the efficacy of bed epilepsy sensors and the merits of the associated telecare service. The evaluation used a number of tools that built on background research involving personal interviews and a postal survey of people with epilepsy and their carers, case studies and consultations with a range of stakeholders. This chapter sets out some of the issues dealt with in the evaluation and places these in a broader context. Verbatim quotes from service users and carers are included to illustrate some of the findings and the views expressed.

Keywords Epilepsy · Seizure · Telecare

1 Description of the Project

The Epilepsy Project (hereafter 'the Project') took place in the Republic of Ireland. It was evaluated with funding from the Irish Government's Enhancing Disability Services Programme, over a period of two years from 2006 to 2008. Particular

M. J. Fisk (✉)
Health Design and Technology Institute, Coventry University Technology Park,
Puma Way, Coventry, CV1 2TT, UK
e-mail: mfisk@cad.coventry.ac.uk

Commun Med Care Compunetics (2011) 3: 15–30
DOI: 10.1007/8754_2011_28
© Springer-Verlag Berlin Heidelberg 2011
Published Online: 14 June 2011

attention in this chapter is given to evaluative work in the latter part of 2007. This related, in the main, to information derived from users, carers and other stakeholders who had, by this time, a relatively long experience of providing or using the bed epilepsy sensors and the related telecare service. The term telecare embraces services that deliver in relation to people's care needs via telecommunications technologies. Both this and subsequent work by the author (and lead evaluator of the Project) regarding the role of bed epilepsy sensors enables their potential to be considered in a wider context. Some issues that have arisen through the mainstreaming of the Project are noted.

Two key agencies were involved in the Project, one a charity concerned for the needs of people with epilepsy and their carers, the other a housing, care, support and telecare service. Respectively the organizations are based in the Republic of Ireland and Northern Ireland but each operate throughout Ireland. Almost all of the users who joined the Project were identified by the charity. They were referred to the Project because of the nature of their seizures and their potential to benefit from the additional support that it was envisaged that the service would give. None of those referred was considered able, except with difficulty, to afford the technology and the monitoring charge for the service in question. The service was provided free of charge for the duration of the Project.

Overall 45 households within which one person had epilepsy had been recruited to the Project by 2008. No charge was made for either the equipment or the service. With mainstreaming now having taken place and charges now being levied, this number has reduced (at December 2010) to 20. In all such households the person with epilepsy was under 65 years of age. In many cases they were children living with one or more parents; in some they were adult dependents with learning disabilities. Most had long-standing epilepsy with 70% (whether adult or child) having had the condition for 6 years or more. Five (22%) had had their epilepsy since birth. A minority of users (39%) normally experienced a warning or 'aura' that signalled their impending seizure and might mean the ability to call out for help or press a pendant radio trigger (normally worn around the neck).

At the core of the Project was the bed epilepsy sensors provided to the adult or child who experienced seizures. The bed epilepsy sensors linked to small transmitters that enabled, when they were activated, signals to be sent to carephones (see below). With the carephones came pendant radio triggers. These were only worn by some users and not, in any instance, by children. A minority of (adult) users were also provided with fall detectors. The relatively small number using the pendant triggers and fall detectors meant that their efficacy was only lightly considered in the evaluation. While clearly useful to some, they are not discussed in this chapter.

Bed epilepsy sensors are normally positioned beneath the mattress of the person who experiences seizures. They take the form of a flexible film, pad, box or panel that is wired to a bedside monitor. The bedside monitor, through its inbuilt intelligence and programming, enables a person's movements in bed to be interpreted and tonic-clonic seizures, formally known as 'grand mal' attacks (characterised by stiffening and jerking) identified. A signal is then sent directly to a receiving device and a response (and assistance) is able to be obtained. Though not included in this Project, we can note that some bed epilepsy sensors can work alongside additional trigger devices such as noise or moisture sensors with both of these providing a further means of signalling that a seizure has commenced. Such other sensors are appropriate for some users, where their seizures are associated with salivation, urination or cries.

In the Project the bed epilepsy sensors linked, via a radio transmitter, to a carephone (also known as a social alarm, safety alarm or personal response system). The carephone, on being triggered by the bed epilepsy device, in turn connects via the telephone network to the telecare monitoring and response centre. The overall system facilitated the kind of response that is now well recognised for many social alarm services that are usually aimed at meeting the support needs of older people. These offer the means by which when a 'call' is received a two-way speech channel is opened. Advice and/or reassurance can be provided; and action, where appropriate, taken to enable help to be given. By virtue of linking to a monitoring and response centre in Northern Ireland from users in the Republic of Ireland, the Project was cross-border—involving separate European countries.

At the point of its initiation, it would have been difficult to overstate the importance of this Project. This follows from the novelty of the technologies concerned and the extent of the support needs, noted below, of many people with epilepsy. No prior (or known subsequent) evaluation of such technologies and an associated service that supports people with epilepsy in their own homes has been undertaken. Issues relating to the technologies and the manner of their operation are noted later in this chapter. But in order to understand the broader context, initial discussion of the needs of some people with epilepsy is necessary.

The first key point to make is that there are estimated to be between 33,000 and 36,000 people aged 5 years or older in the Republic of Ireland being treated for epilepsy [1]. The same research points to the prevalence rate (the number of people with epilepsy per 1000 in the overall population) in the Republic of Ireland being in keeping with other parts of Europe at 8.3–9 per 1000 in 2005. There is a marginally higher prevalence rate for men than women and the rate increases with age. The prevalence rate is increasing. There is, however, substantial misdiagnosis of epilepsy, noted by the Joint Epilepsy Council of the UK and Ireland as between 20 and 31%. Additionally, there are concerns in many member countries of the European Union regarding the extent of delays in treatment for people with suspected or diagnosed epilepsy [2].

The relatively high rate of misdiagnosis for epilepsy is a matter of considerable concern. It arises, in large part, from the absence of a test for epilepsy; the fact that there are many types of seizure; and the inconvenient fact that people who experience seizures cannot be their own witnesses except for what they remember in the periods before and after the event. In this Project the concern was to use bed epilepsy sensors to support people with epilepsy who experienced just tonic-clonic seizures. Other seizures not associated with the same degree of movement (e.g. 'absence seizures' where there is a loss of attention and disorientation) cannot be readily identified by devices that are unattached to the body.

The second key point to make is that when a tonic-clonic seizure occurs the person is likely to need urgent assistance in order for the administration of 'rescue' medication (normally diazepam) as a calmer. Such medication is normally administered anally—through other options are becoming available. It requires, therefore, the privacy that is normally associated with a person's home and the help of a known carer, likely to be a family member. The carer will also provide the person with re-assurance as they recover from what was inevitably a stressful experience. There can, in addition, sometimes be the need for treatment arising from injury as a result of a fall.

The urgency of the need for treatment becomes even clearer when the possibility of SUDEP (sudden death through epilepsy) is taken into account. SUDEP arises where tonic-clonic seizures are repeated or prolonged over a period of about half an hour—in a condition known as status epilepticus. Ninety-one cases were reported by general practitioners of 'probable or definite' SUDEP in the Republic of Ireland in the five year period from 2000 [3].

The third key point is the fact that epilepsy, especially when associated with tonic-clonic seizures, carries a stigma. The stigma relates to the fears (and often lack of understanding) of other people about epilepsy; its association with learning disability (where there is a high prevalence of epilepsy); and the natural embarrassment that someone with epilepsy feels through the loss of control of their bodies. This stigma is acutely felt by most people with the condition. And given the unpredictability of the onset of seizures, it is not unsurprising that there are associated anxieties. The combined effect of that stigma and anxiety means that many people with the condition, are inhibited about or are (in the case of driving) precluded from participating in the 'normal' activities of economic and social life. A degree of social exclusion is, therefore, a commonplace consequence. Social exclusion may also be a fact of life for carers given the continuity (and often intensity) of the care that many provide for people with epilepsy.

A study of epilepsy patients of Cork University Hospital in the Republic of Ireland, it can be noted, found a clear correlation between the extent of stigma felt by people with epilepsy with the severity of the seizures that they experienced. This was reflected in people's strategies of concealment of their condition in order to appear to conform to accepted 'social norms' [4]. The association of epilepsy with anxiety was noted in a more recent review [5].

Following from all the above, it is axiomatic that a tonic-clonic seizure, however identified, must be regarded as a potential emergency. Hence there is a strong argument for further exploration of the role and efficacy of bed epilepsy sensors. There is also a necessity for an eye to be kept on further technological developments that might afford support to people with or help in the diagnosis and treatment of the condition. Initially, however, we can consider the role of bed epilepsy sensors in facilitating a response to 'events' as, perhaps, a natural candidate for inclusion with other aspects of digital homecare and as having something in common with fall detectors and with what was seen as a primary purpose of conventional social alarms [6].

Finally, lest there be any predisposition among some to consider people with epilepsy as a single group with similar needs, the variability in the nature and frequency of seizures must be reaffirmed. There are additional support needs of some people whose epilepsy is associated with learning disability, stroke or acquired brain injury. The foregoing adds substantially to the challenge of addressing the needs of people with epilepsy in the context of digital homecare.

The above issues position the Project in the Republic of Ireland as one concerned, therefore, with an aspect of digital homecare that has not been explored elsewhere. It relates to a significant population that stands to benefit from the same.

2 Development of the Project

Development of the Project examined in this chapter was in part facilitated through the established expertise of the telecare service provider. This telecare service now links over 20,000 household throughout Ireland. Most of the service users (in excess of 95%) are older people. The organisation was (and remains), however, very conscious of broader potential of telecare and is at the forefront of initiatives that are operationalising new ways of working at the health and social care interface. The rapid development of new technologies (including bed epilepsy sensors) they saw as offering tools that could underpin services for a 'new' group of users. Importantly they could provide the service in a way that could potentially empower users and enable them to live more independently.

That the Project should focus on people with epilepsy related to the shared sense of inquiry (of both the key organisations involved) regarding bed epilepsy sensors that were, in 2006, 'new arrivals' onto the telecare market. Significantly by this time, the sensors were, through the use of radio transmitters, able to be linked to carephones. Stand-alone bed epilepsy sensors with local alerts for seizures (through e.g. the use of buzzers and pagers) had, however, been available for some 3–4 years prior.

With regard to service users, the evaluation of the Project was primarily based information from survey respondents among the 45 households who were part of the same by the autumn of 2008. This included ten households who had joined the Project in the preceding year. Thirty-five of the households can be described as adults with epilepsy; the other ten being children or young adults who were substantially dependent on an adult parent. Service users were spread throughout the Republic of Ireland, with some concentration in the Dublin and Cork areas. Personal interviews with 6 service users undertaken in August 2007 were supplemented by a postal survey of the remaining 39. Allowing for non-responses, engagement took place with 23 users (or their carers in the case of children or adults with learning disabilities). This represented half (51%) of the total households that were part of the service.

The aims and objectives of the Project were, for people with epilepsy, to

- identify the need for and provide support for their independent living;
- promote their self-confidence and well-being; and
- explore the effectiveness of the technologies as a means of identifying their epileptic seizures.

Accompanying these aims and objectives was a series of challenging questions posed that related to people's views of and understandings of the sensors, the way that they used them, their impact on the risks to which they were exposed, and their satisfaction with the both the sensors and the telecare service of which they were part.

The personal interviews and postal survey noted above were supplemented through secondary research, by case studies and by consultation with various stakeholders. The secondary research focused more broadly on the experiences and needs of people with epilepsy. Only to a limited extent (a matter dictated by the scarcity of such information) was there a focus on the technologies themselves and their potential within the broader context of telecare. More detail of the Project framework, the methodology adopted and Project outcomes have been published elsewhere [7].

3 Outcomes

For the most part, the outcomes of the Project were such that the aims and objectives noted above were satisfied. Much was revealed in the evaluation about the value that came to be placed on the bed epilepsy sensors provided (and the related telecare service) by users (and their carers) and by the various stakeholders who were witness to the benefits. There were also very useful pointers in the evaluation as to how people felt about the technology and, crucially, how in many cases they felt empowered by it. Nevertheless, for a small minority there were negative experiences. Important lessons can be learnt from these.

Of note with regard to users (and their carers) it is clear that there was a high degree of acceptance of the technologies. This followed initial decisions by users (or carers) to join the Project based on the expected opportunities that the technologies would provide. No figures are available regarding the number of people initially approached but who decided not to join the Project. And while there will, for any Project, be some turnover of users it is noteworthy that just four out of an initial 39 users left the service in the 12 months that followed the first phase. As noted below, further losses have taken place since the Project (and, therefore, cost-free provision) ended.

Some of the most relevant outcomes are dealt with more fully later in this chapter when user aspects are addressed. At this stage it can be noted that there were both psychological and practical benefits for both users and carers that derived from the sensors and the service, with each contributing to an overall improvement in well-being.

Most survey respondents reported that they regarded the devices as having a positive effect on their lives. All but one of the adult users reported 'feeling safer' by virtue of having the bed epilepsy sensor in their home. And a near unanimity of response was evident in relation to the statement 'I/my child can live more independently with telecare devices'.

> Prior to having the alarms we had no way of knowing that he was having a seizure. Now we can get to him quickly.
>
> I find it very beneficial as at least now I can stay with my child during a seizure instead of running around looking for a phone! My child feels better because I don't have to leave him.
>
> Immediate assistance keeps seizure time to a minimum—with the use of emergency medication
>
> [The service] gives us more confidence and a sense of security—help is at hand.

The overall positive outcomes are reflected in the extent to which service users were retained after project completion. At this point, what was a free service became subject to a charge of €30 or €50 per calendar month. The higher charge included provision of a fall detector in addition to the bed epilepsy sensor. In both cases the charge covered the link to a carephone and the provision of the monitoring and response service.

In all, as at December 2010, 18 of the original 45 service users were retained. The retention of seven of these (five at the higher level) was thanks to funding made by local offices of the Irish Health Service Executive based on an assessment of need. The remaining 11 pay for the service themselves. Ten of the 11 in question pay for just the minimum level of service—this reflecting the fact that their initial referral to the Project had been based on both need and their inability to pay, except with difficulty, for the service.

Some people will, of course, have been 'lost' to the service as a result of changing family circumstances and/or a diminution in need (perhaps because the seizures were now controlled). Anecdotal information, however, points to many having left the service because they could not afford it. With this in mind, therefore, the level of retention is considered to be a genuine indication of the fact that a real need was being satisfied by the technologies and the service.

It can be noted, in addition, that there is some growth (12 by December 2010) in the number of new users of bed epilepsy sensors provided through the service— these meeting the needs of people living in their own homes and, through charitable organisations, in specialist accommodation. Such growth has followed the heightened awareness of the merits of bed epilepsy sensors among staff within the lead organisations and a number of specialist epilepsy nurses who had had contact with the Project.

With regard to the recommendations that emerged from the evaluation, these included the need for further development of working practices that were already being demonstrated viz. partnership working between agencies and the provision of good information about the technologies and related service. Other recommendations related to operational and a technical issues that are discussed later in this chapter. The operational issue was concerned to ensure (in a context where the need for speedy responses to had to be recognised) that alerts should not necessarily be required to go through the monitoring and response centre in Northern Ireland—but rather that local alerts (with the monitoring centre as 'back up') would be in many instances appropriate. The technical issue relating to sensitivity levels was such that a recommendation was made for representations to be made to the manufacturer that related to design improvements—whereby adjustments to sensitivity might be able to be made without necessitating a home visit by engineers.

With regard to the issue of local alerts it is now the norm for the service that carers are alerted directly (through e.g. a call to a mobile phone) when a seizure is identified. Users, however, have opted to retain the link to the monitoring and response centre as 'back up'. This clearly reflects shared understandings of the importance of speedy responses to tonic-clonic seizures when they occur. With regard to the facility for adjusting sensitivity, the matter was drawn to the attention of the equipment suppliers but, to date, what was considered a shortcoming in design remains.

4 Internal Influences on Development and Outcome

The fact that the Project was utilising a novel technology meant that it was essential for all parties to be included within the evaluation process. It follows that the focus of the evaluation would embrace both the personal experience of the users (and their carers) in terms of their interaction with and use of the technologies; and the impact (practical and psychological) that the technologies had on them.

Consultation also took place with stakeholders among who were healthcare practitioners (including a consultant neurologist and specialist epilepsy nurses) and an academic. Their responses revealed a strong sense of enquiry but in a context where none had prior experience of bed epilepsy sensors, fall detectors or telecare services. They had no preconceptions, therefore, regarding likely benefits of the technologies and had been guided by (and learnt from) the two lead organisations regarding their likely potential. The role of the healthcare staff during the course of the evaluation remained unchanged except that their contact with users (their patients) would necessarily encompass consideration with them of the way in which the bed epilepsy sensors and the related telecare service were or were not of practical or psychological benefit.

Consultees from the service provider revealed their focus as less to do with clinical benefits (a matter that was outside their remit) and more to do with well-being and supporting independent living at home—contributing, therefore, to 'digital homecare'. They were, however, responsible for the provision, installation and calibration of the bed epilepsy sensors in the homes of the users through a network of installers. Consultation with those installers as part of the evaluation made clear the extent to which this required good interpersonal skills and patience on their part. And it is pertinent to note that, as well as undertaking the technical tasks, the installers provided users (including carers) with information about and guidance regarding the operation of the devices. They had, furthermore, to set the sensitivity levels and invariably made one or more revisits in order for an optimum level, in relation to the needs of individual users, to be established.

The importance of correctly setting the sensitivity levels for bed epilepsy sensors cannot be easily overstated. The levels will need to be higher or lower depending on the size and weight of the user and the characteristics of their seizures. Adjustments might also be required to the positioning of the sensor (in relation to the body movements associated with the seizure pattern) or to provide re-enforcement below soft and springy mattresses.

The objective, in setting the sensitivity level, was to 'capture' all tonic-clonic seizures (with a signal then being sent to the carephone) but at the same time to minimise the number of false alarms. A further adjustment, it should be noted, was possible regarding the time delay before an alert was sent—this facilitating cancellation of any false alarms by the user (or carer) before a link to the monitoring and response centre was made.

> Her siblings worry when it is activated accidentally as they fear she is having a seizure when she is not.
>
> The bed sensor is too sensitive. I'm always conscious of setting it off—dashing to cancel the call.

The only other known evaluation of bed epilepsy sensors (in a New York hospital setting rather than in people's homes) illustrates well the point regarding sensitivity [8]. The New York study used a bed epilepsy sensor from a different manufacturer to that used in the Project that is the subject of this chapter. The study was focused on the monitoring of 64 hospital patients from midnight to 8 a.m. over (in total) a period of 1528 h. In that period the devices successfully identified five out of the eight tonic clonic seizures that were known to have occurred. There were, however, 269 false alarms (i.e. 'false positives' where an alert was sent but there was no seizure). Such a high level of false alarms can be regarded as excessive. We can speculate that a higher sensitivity setting on the bed epilepsy sensor and/or better positioning in relation to any particular pattern of seizure, would have meant all the tonic-clonic seizures being identified, but a price would have been likely to have been paid in terms of an even higher rate of false alarms. Despite such issues the study concluded that there is a role for such devices. It called for further study 'ideally in a home setting'.

For the Project that is focused on in this chapter, the expectation placed on the 45 users (or their carers) was simply that they should be willing, in personal interviews or through the postal survey, to report on their experience. In so doing the service providers saw the users as helping in the development of a rounded understanding of the potential (or otherwise) of bed epilepsy sensors and the appropriateness, for this user group, of their use within a telecare service. As has been noted, users played their part and did so in relation to either their own positions as adults with epilepsy or as carers of children or carers of adult dependents with learning disabilities.

5 External Influences on Development and Outcome

There were few external influences on the Project except for those that reflected a growing understanding among professionals and others of the need for improved services for people with epilepsy. The Project simply represented, therefore, one way in which a telecare service could extend its role to embrace people of all ages.

Telecare services in Ireland were (and remain) few in number and are very much focused on the needs of older people. Service developments in Northern Ireland (where the monitoring service is located) were, however, increasingly being influenced by the changing pattern of provision in other parts of the United Kingdom. In the UK there was a predisposition to use a widening range of sensors and peripheral devices linking to carephones; and a trend towards a widening role of services to ones that were less focused on the needs of (or specialist provision for) older people.

There was, in common with other telecare initiatives, some broader consciousness of potential cost savings that might be made through the Project, but this was seen by the lead organisations as a side issue compared with the overriding need to improve services for people with epilepsy. The areas where the service providers recognised the potential for a reduction of costs related, in the main, to the following things.

Firstly, it was considered that the bed epilepsy sensors would facilitate earlier interventions and the appropriate and timely administration of medication. The user would, therefore, benefit from

- better control of his/her seizures;
- a reduction in his/her risk of injury or death;
- a reduced likelihood of hospital admission; and
- his/her better ability to maintain normal life as a parent, employee, etc.

Carers would, at the same time benefit from

- reduced anxiety;
- being able to get more sleep; and (similarly)
- their better ability to maintain normal life as a parent, employee, etc.

The simple point regarding carers being able to get more sleep needs to be emphasised. The evaluation encountered several carers who slept in the same room as the person with epilepsy (often an adult with learning disabilities or a child) in order to be there if he/she had a seizure. All such carers shared a fear of not being alert to a seizure and of being unable, therefore, to provide rescue medication (with all the consequent risks) or to provide reassurance.

To know the telecare service team is there night and day is invaluable.

It is vitally important that our son is empowered to live in his own home. These sensors can help.

[The service] has taken away the fear of my children being taken away from me because of the amount of seizures I was having.

The above means that users and carers stand to gain a sense of greater well-being and, as a direct consequence, are likely to place fewer demands on health and social care services. Importantly (and having an impact on the extent of their social inclusion), users and carers may be more able to maintain a normal family, economic and social life. There can be associated cost savings to the provider agencies. And there can be increased family income and a reduction in the risk of welfare dependency.

Finally, for a few users (or their carers), a potential benefit was observed by virtue of the provision of information (recorded at the monitoring and response centre) about the frequency and timing of their seizures. This information was being used to help clinicians to make diagnoses. This, of course, has benefits in terms of the effectiveness of treatments and potential reductions in the number of hospital admissions and the length of (often expensive) hospital stays.

> [It has provided us with] a monitor of (actual) seizure activity

Legal issues were not addressed in the Project evaluation. By virtue of the Project being provided within the framework of a telecare service, the bed epilepsy sensors were not seen as presenting any legal questions that required to be answered. The sensors were regarded simply as tools to help support independence. By virtue of their not having any connection with the body, they could not be construed as higher level medical devices and they did not warrant, therefore, approvals for use beyond those that related e.g. to their electrical safety and the use of approved radio frequencies. Manufacturers of such devices we can note are, in any case, cautious not to make claims that extend beyond that of their function to monitor movement in a way that can identify patterns that might be associated with seizures. Indeed, most bed epilepsy sensors are presented and marketed as 'movement detectors'.

There were no significant technical developments around bed epilepsy sensors during the period of the Project or since. New models of the devices have not (by January 2011) emerged onto the market and those that are available carry, seemingly, the same functionality—albeit that the algorithms for identifying seizures will be different and subject to adjustments in light of the experience of manufacturers and suppliers with their users. This position is likely to change, however, as greater interest develops in exploring seizure monitoring both for users when in bed and 'on the move'.

6 User Aspects

Broad outcomes of the Project have been signalled earlier in this chapter relating to a general assertion of the benefits of bed epilepsy sensors and the related telecare service. Indeed, around four out of every five respondents (82%) to the personal interviews and postal survey regarded the devices as having a positive effect on their lives. We must note, however, that two respondents (8%) felt the devices a 'mixed blessing' with both positive and negative aspects; and one respondent felt the effect was altogether negative.

The negativity in question related, in two cases, to number and frequency of false alerts and their impact on carers. These represented an inconvenience—with the bed epilepsy sensors therefore failing (albeit after attempts to find the optimum level of sensitivity or time delay before alerts being sent) to give the carer the better quality of life they had hoped for. In the third case the inconvenience arose because of the regularity by which the carer was being alerted because of the 'type of continuous seizures' experienced by her daughter. She had given the bed epilepsy sensor and carephone back.

> At her [daughter's] worst the alarm was going off every two minutes … [I was] running in and out continuously. I found it was more of a bother than a help

The negative responses in the evaluation were, however, outweighed by positive ones. Typical of several carers was the reporting of one parent (reflecting a point made earlier in this chapter) who described how the devices had provided her with 'peace of mind' since she does not need to check on her daughter at regular intervals throughout the night. She reported, therefore, that she could now sleep more easily knowing that she will be wakened if the need arose. But counterbalancing this benefit she observed that accidental activation of the sensor is frightening and confusing both to her and her daughter.

Another parent mentioned how she had had eight months of sleep deprivation because she was so worried about her son's nocturnal seizures. She said that the devices made her feel more relaxed and she now sleeps better because she knows the devices will alert her. A further parent reported that her son (with severe cognitive disabilities) was less anxious because he knew that every time he has a seizure, somebody would come to him. Prior to the installation of devices, he was unable to raise the alarm himself because of his disabilities.

> [The service makes] a huge impact on our home environment. I can now get some real sleep at night and know I will be alerted automatically if my son needs assistance. Thank you

The overall context is one, therefore, in which a clear majority of users and carers, albeit with some concerns about the technical efficacy (around sensitivity and false alarms), view bed epilepsy sensors with favour. This was reflected in a clear majority feeling that the devices were 'useful' or 'very useful'. Only in one case did a parent feel that the epilepsy sensor was 'not useful'.

With regard to quality of life, the evaluation reported that close to half (53%) of respondents affirmed that this had improved since they, or their dependent, had had the bed epilepsy sensor. For some others, the evaluation reported that while their quality of life may not have changed, the devices did provide them with greater re-assurance and offered them at least the potential to maintain the quality of life that they had.

All but one (93%) of the adult users reported 'feeling safer' by virtue of having the bed epilepsy sensor in their home. Two-thirds strongly agreed with the statement 'I feel much safer'. The evaluation noted that this feeling of being safer was more emphatically reported than in previous interviews and in the outcomes of a postal survey undertaken in the first phase of the evaluation (during 2006). The difference, albeit relating to small numbers, was suggested as being explained by the ability of users to assess the merits of the bed epilepsy sensor over a longer period. Similarly reflecting a positive user experience, the evaluation reported a near unanimity of response (86%) in relation to the statement 'I/my child can live more independently with telecare devices'—again expressed more emphatically than in the first phase of the evaluation.

All but two of the respondents (90%) were reported as being happy with the service they received from the monitoring and response centre. For the two who stated that they were not happy, the evaluation reported this as resulting from miscommunication and/or misunderstandings between the service user and the service provider. The latter may have related, it was suggested, to the view expressed by some respondents (notably carers) regarding the lack of necessity for calls to be made to the monitoring and response centre in Northern Ireland when they were (for instance) located in the next room. As noted earlier, this matter has now been addressed.

The experience of bed epilepsy sensors was, therefore, a positive one for most users and carers. Following from this, and in the interest of sharing knowledge and learning lessons from the Project, three cameos (drawn from longer case studies) are offered that illustrate different user (and carer) perspectives. All the names are changed to maintain confidentiality.

Jane, aged 37

Jane lives with her two sons. She has had epilepsy for over 10 years. Her tonic-clonic seizures occur once or twice a week, with some seizures repeatedly occurring over two or three days. She has the bed epilepsy sensor installed; she wears the pendant transmitter and a fall detector.

Jane feels that the devices have been of great benefit to her as she is at home on her own with the children. Sometimes her seizures leave her unaware of her surroundings for up to 3 h. She used to worry about what would happen to her sons but now has a greater sense of (both her and their) security. This is especially the case now her eldest son knows how the devices work and can play a part in getting help for his mother.

Jane's use of the bed epilepsy sensor illustrates very clearly their role in supporting normal family life. Her sons, though increasing in their understanding and ability to help their mother, are reassured by the fact that help and support can be obtained quickly.

Richard, aged 9

Richard has had epilepsy since he was a baby and has the bed epilepsy sensor installed. He has regular simple partial and tonic-clonic seizures that last between 30 s and two minutes.

His mother had little sleep in the 8 months before the sensor was fitted. She reported that the devices helped the whole family to sleep and feel more relaxed. While a little concerned that false alarms were caused by her young children 'jumping on the bed' she said that the response from the staff (at the monitoring centre) was 'brilliant'.

Richard's use of the epilepsy sensor illustrates a major benefit to the life of his mother through the 'simple' fact that she can sleep peacefully, knowing that she will be alerted if he has a seizure.

> Brendan, aged 29
>   Brendan has had epilepsy for over 10 years and has frequent, usually nocturnal, tonic-clonic seizures. He lives with his mother. He feels 'safe and secure' with the carephone and pendant, bed epilepsy sensor and fall detector, these enabling him to maintain a record of his seizures that help when he sees his neurologist.
>   Brendan's concern is the sensitivity of the bed sensor. This was adjusted, but then it was not going off when a seizure was occurring. He would like the technologies to be developed to be less sensitive but still effective for seizures.

Brendan's use of the epilepsy sensor illustrates the potential for recording his seizures and using the information in reviews of his medication and in understanding his condition.

The user aspects indicated and illustrated in part by the cameos, point to a minimal need on the part of many users (and carers) for education or training regarding the bed epilepsy sensors and their role. In any case, the users and carers mostly have expert knowledge of epilepsy and the characteristics of the seizures experienced. The evaluation pointed, furthermore, to their being ready to take on new knowledge that related to their participation in the Project.

7 General Aspects

The Project examined in this chapter is important by virtue of it being the only one known to examine the efficacy of bed epilepsy sensors as a contributor to supporting independent living for a particular range of potential beneficiaries. A relatively wide range of potential users (adults, children, people with learning disabilities) was embraced, but it must be recognised that people aged over 65 were not included.

What was striking from the evaluation of the Project was the extent to which, unlike other telecare applications, the benefits of the bed epilepsy sensors are both to the users and the carers. In the case of the former a clear and major benefit was expressed regarding the fact that help could be obtained and even people's lives can be saved. The ability of bed epilepsy sensors to alert people of a seizure occurring appears, therefore have been the primary benefit. Arising from this, however, is the reassurance to the user and his/her carers—with, in most cases, an added bonus for both arising in their quality of life.

> If I suffered status epilepticus again it would probably save my life
>   If I'm on my own I feel more safe because of the alarm

As an aspect of digital homecare, therefore, an interesting application of a new technology has been demonstrated by the Project. It is one, furthermore, where the extent of need has been indicated as being substantial and one where further technological developments relating to seizure identification and the obtaining of help can be anticipated.

Given the above it was important that the lessons learnt should be disseminated. Such dissemination has taken place through the delivery by the author of this chapter of four seminar and conference presentations; and through articles in academic and professional journals [7, 9].

8 Conclusion

The needs of and issues facing people with epilepsy and their carers in the context of digital homecare have not, aside from in relation to the limited number of publications and papers regarding the Project (noted above), previously been addressed. This is despite the availability of bed epilepsy sensors and their growing use both outside and within telecare services. This lack of attention in part relates to the fact that such devices remain little known.

The efficacy of bed epilepsy devices is, however, signaled in the Project reported on in this chapter. And given the extent of need within the Republic of Ireland and beyond, further use and development of such technologies will undoubtedly take place. That further development, it is clear from the Project and from the New York hospital based study [7, 8], must give attention to the issue of sensitivity and/or the sophistication of the algorithms by which seizures are identified from the complex range of body movements that are monitored. This means the assuredness by which (at least) tonic-clonic seizures are identified will increase while the rate of false alarms is reduced—potentially delivering even greater benefits to users of the devices (and carers) and associated telecare or related services.

The evaluation we can note as reporting the Project in Ireland as having met its key aims and objectives. Support for independent living and the promotion of well-being (for users and carers) were demonstrated. Certainly the basic aim of demonstrating the efficacy of bed epilepsy sensors as providing a means of identifying at least tonic-clonic seizures was fulfilled. Problems that were encountered were offset by the very positive experience of most users and carers. Of further significance, however, is the indication, in the Project, of the potential of the technologies to provide some help in the process of diagnosis—e.g. through gathering and maintaining a record of information regarding frequency and timing of a person's seizures.

Sensors that relate to the needs of people with epilepsy will, therefore, remain part of the range of technological options available to people within telecare services and ipso facto of digital homecare. This chapter gives an initial pointer to their effectiveness in an Irish context and alerts the reader to technological developments to come.

Finally, in the context of the wider range of digital homecare initiatives, the Project gives welcome attention to the role of technologies that respond to a need that affect adults and children of all ages. It is a useful reminder, therefore, for service providers to consider technologies according to such need rather than according to age.

References

1. Linehan C, Kerr MP, Walsh PN, Brady G, Kelleher C, Delany N, Dawson F, Glynn M. Examining the prevalence of epilepsy and delivery of epilepsy care in Ireland. Epilepsia. 2010;51(5):845–52.
2. Joint Epilepsy Council of the UK and Ireland. Epilepsy: The Consequencies of Inadequate Health and Education Services. Leeds; 2010.
3. O'Rourke D. National Study on Sudden Unexpected Death in Epilepsy. Dublin: Brainwave—The Irish Epilepsy Association.
4. Ni Eidhin MN, McLeavey B. The relationship between perceived acceptance, stigma and severity in a population with epilepsy. Ir J Psychol. 2001;22(3–4):213–22.
5. Baker G, Eatock J. Epilepsy and anxiety. Epilepsy Prof. 2007;6:31–3.
6. Fisk MJ. Social alarms to telecare: older people's services in transition. Bristol: The Policy Press; 2003.
7. Fisk M. Indicated benefits of bed epilepsy sensors to users of a telecare service in the Republic of Ireland. J Assist Technol. 2009;37–40.
8. Carlson C, Arnedo V, Cahill M, Devinsky O. Detecting nocturnal convulsions: efficacy of the MP5 Monitor. Seizure. 2009;18:225–7.
9. Fisk M. Bed epilepsy sensors. Epilepsy Prof. 2009;14:34–35.

The Videocommunication to Support Care Delivery to Independently Living Seniors

Charles G. Willems, Marieke D. Spreeuwenberg, Loek A. van der Heide, Luc P. de Witte and John Rietman

Abstract Demographic trends in southern Netherlands predict an increasing aging population in the next decade. There will not be enough health care providers available to meet the growing demand of care of elderly. Therefore, there is a need to reorganize the Dutch health care system in a more efficient way. In this process, innovative technologies can play an important role. Videocommunication enables elderly living at home to contact the health care organization by a 24/7 screen-to-screen video communication. Several care organizations started projects to implement videocommunication. Different combinations of technology were used, ranging from high speed remote controlled cameras combined with a set top box connected to a regular TV set, to a webcam using a computer based internet application. These experiments were enabled by grants from the Dutch government to support the investment by care organizations, as well as an experimental provision to arrange for the re-imbursement of the services. The introduction of videocommunication was accompanied by a monitor to clarify the progress made at client level as well as organizational level. In this paper a description of the developments between 2005 and 2010 will be given. From the introduction of videocommunication in the Netherlands, the authors of this paper have been working together to develop and implement videocommunication in a Dutch health care organization active in the province of Limburg the aim of this implementation project is to apply videocommunication to enable older people to live longer independently at home

C. G. Willems · M. D. Spreeuwenberg · L. A. van der Heide
L. P. de Witte
Zuyd University, PO. Box 550, 6400 AN Heerlen, The Netherlands
e-mail: c.g.m.h.willems@hszuyd.nl

J. Rietman (✉)
Proteion Thuis, PO. Box 218, 5800 AE Venray, The Netherlands
e-mail: johnrietman@proteion.nl

Commun Med Care Compunetics (2011) 3: 31–42
DOI: 10.1007/8754_2011_21
© Springer-Verlag Berlin Heidelberg 2011
Published Online: 25 May 2011

in a responsible and safe manner. A longitudinal study was conducted with 124 frail elderly clients of the home care organization. A regionally based communication infrastructure was organized to handle alerts and incoming messages from the elderly. A questionnaire was used to measure the clients' feelings of loneliness and feelings of safety at baseline level and after 1 year (April 2010). Protocols for implementation and educational material have been developed to support organizations in the implementation of videocommunication. Applied research has been done at development level as well as implementation level of new applications and communication infrastructure supported by videocommunication. This paper, will shown how the introduction of videocommunication was carried out by the home-care organization. Information will be given on the development of services like a "Good morning, Good evening" service. The aim of this services is to provide daily structure, support of compliance with medication intake and prevention of social isolation by means of screen-to-screen videocommunication. Developments of consultation by means of videocommunication with a general practitioner and an application to facilitate memory training are currently under development and will be discussed. In the study almost all clients indicate that their feeling of loneliness has increased by the system. They feel that there is always someone who takes care for them which has a real positive impact on the clients. However, technical problems with the system still occur and finding a sustainable financial structure is a challenge.

Keywords Videocommunication · Care · Evaluation of use

1 Description of the Project

The participating organization is a home-care organization active in the province of Limburg. It delivers home care support to persons living in their own environment. As in all western countries, in this region the organization is confronted with a double demographic shift; a graying of the population causes an increase in care demand. Also, in the mid-term perspective, a reduction in workforce is to be expected. These two developments are accompanied by budgetary restrictions. Together, this indicates that within foreseeable time it will not be possible to continue service delivery in the situation as it stands. This consideration stimulated the management of the care organization to look for the development of alternatives. It is noted that in many research projects technological developments are identified as potential solution, yet technical organizational and ethical issues need to be addressed [1]. In home care delivery an essential part of the service delivery process is supported by communication between clients and care providers. Modern communication technology techniques enable the simultaneous use of video and voice communication which can even be distributed throughout a regular TV. Videocommunication may also become supportive to homecare workers themselves. It can serve as an easy accessible feedback system, while being active in an ambulant way for instance by consulting a colleague or by getting access to patient files on a remote way. Moreover, videocommunication may support the self management of care for chronic patients by giving relevant information on what to do in critical situations or by supporting the improvement of the lifestyle. These arguments stimulated the management of the care organization to investigate the potentials of videocommunication as a supportive tool for care delivery in future.

2 Development of the Project

The analysis of future developments resulted in the decision of the care organization to start an experiment using videocommunication. In the period 2004–2006 several companies in the Netherlands were able to provide the technical means to support videocommunication on an already existing platform in the house. The advantage of this approach is that the client is already acquainted to the use of this apparatus. Furthermore, the use of this technology enabled the use of technology communication protocols like ISDN and ADSL. It was expected that the use of this approach may lead to a cost effective solution, since only minor investments in the hardware infrastructure were needed.

It was expected that clients would prefer this way of videocommunication prior to the use of computer mediated communication approaches, simply because of the fact that they are familiar with the use of a TV set. The use of videocommunication is a new approach. Traditionally, communication between the homecare organization and their clients is done either by the use of a telephone or through direct contact done either in an office or at the client's home. The use of videocommunication as a means of the care delivery at a distance urges the care organization, the care workers and the clients to re-establish their expectations and procedures.

The care organization first started a pilot to deliver videocommunication to a selection of their clients. This was done to see whether it is technically possible to set up the requirements needed for a larger project. Also the initial reactions of clients and care workers to the new required procedures was tested. A total of 20 clients was reached. At the end of this small scale pilot the management decided to set up a bigger, more ambitious project. The idea of this project (described in detail in this paper) is to organize a prolonged period of use and to setup a monitor to determine several aspects, which are: client expectations and satisfaction, effects on feelings of loneliness and safety, the actual use of applications delivered by videocommunication, the willingness of clients to pay for these services, identification of future needs in applications and the actual process of service delivery. In Fig. 1 a screenshot is shown of the actual image of the videocommunication screen.

Fig. 1 Screenshot of the
actual image of the
videocommunication

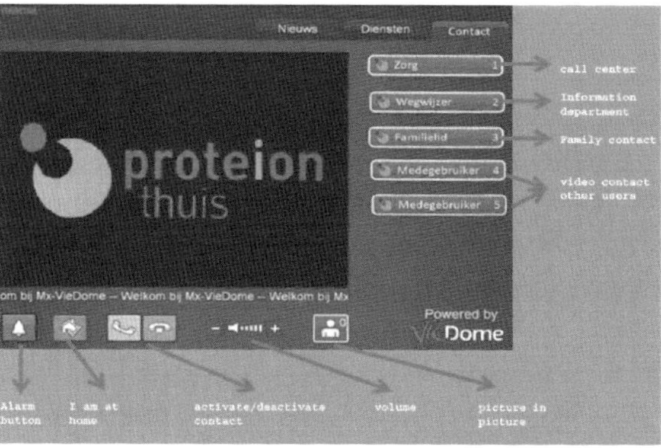

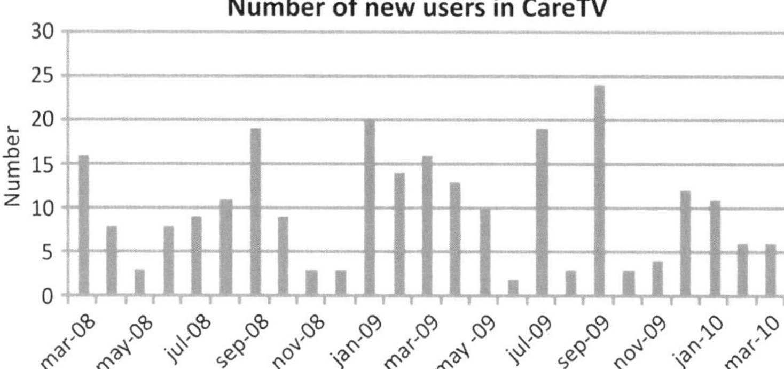

Fig. 2 Number of new participants using the videocommunication

3 Outcome of the Project

By applying an extensive monitor, the use of videocommunication was monitored
over a period of 2 years [2]. During this period 201 clients used the videocommunication. The attraction of new clients was done through marketing activities
performed by trained care workers who have regular contact with existing clients.
Moreover, corporate communication activities were performed, which were: pre-
paring brochures, creating a website and organizing publications in local newspa-
pers. Due to the experimental stage of the project, clients did not have to pay for this
service, they could accept this service as an extra since their regular service would
continue. Once the clients decided to participate they were included in the monitor
activities. In Fig. 2 the actual entry of clients is shown. The entry of new clients
expressed in numbers per month varied from 2 up to 24. This fluctuation could, to
some degree, be explained by the intensity of efforts made to attract new clients. For
instance, in the month preceding January 2009 and September 2009 intensive

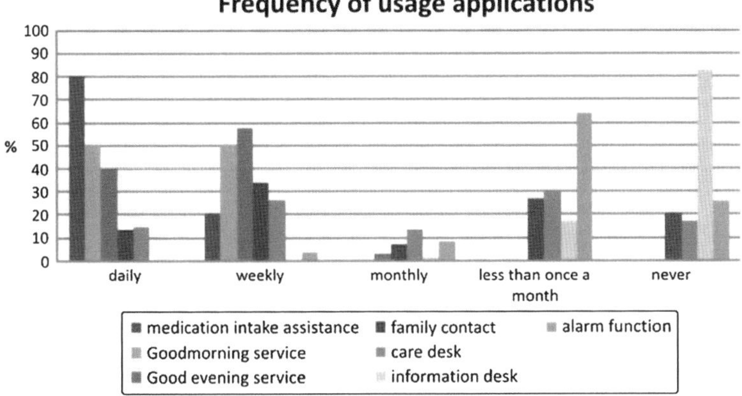

Fig. 3 Frequency of usage of the applications of the videocommunication

Table 1 Average use of the videocommunication per client per month

Period	Number of clients	Minutes care TV	Average minutes per client
November 2008	32	570	18
April 2009	63	2317	36
October 2009	70	3051	44
March 2010	105	4553	43

communication was performed towards the care workers of the care organization as part of the preparation of an instruction meeting. Being introduced to the potentials of the videocommunication themselves, they were stimulated to communicate about the potential benefits of Care TV with their clients. 102 clients participated in a monitor in which at a 6 month interval measurements were performed of actual use, expectations and user satisfaction. The results show (Fig. 3) that the medication and the Good Morning Good Evening service GMGA) are used on a daily basis, whereas the alarm function is used less than once per month.

The average use of the videocommunication measured as a sum of all applications changes from a total of 15 min per client in 2008 to 43 min per client in April 2010. In Table 1 the average use of the videocommunication is given.

The results in Table 1 indicate that there is a steady increase of new clients and consequently the use of the videocommunication expressed as total minutes increases. User satisfaction was measured as well, yet this does not hold for all the individual services. In Fig. 4 the number of clients and the average time of contacts are given for the GMGA service.

The results clearly show that the average time of contact decreases drastically. The reason for this decrease may be a reflection of the pressure care workers involved in the delivery of GMGA experienced during the study period. An increase in demand resulted in an increase of their workload. Most of the contacts through the GMGA application were considered to be "social talk". These contacts could be

Fig. 4 Use of GMGA
expressed as number of
clients and average time of
contact expressed as minutes
per client

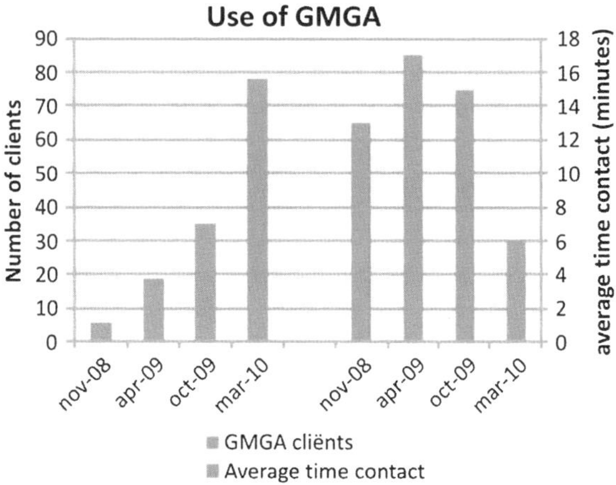

Fig. 5 Example of the
videocommunication

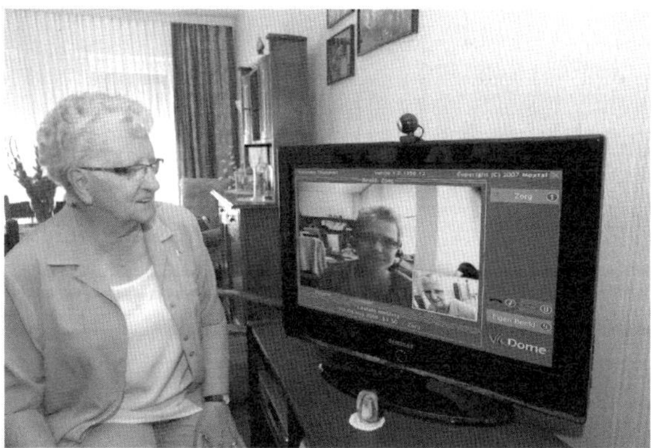

either initiated by the client or were started by the care worker based on a regular
appointment to do so. Clients using GMGA often used this service on a daily basis,
this in contrast to the alarm or information service. In Fig. 5. an example of the
active videocommunication is presented.

The results at client level indicate that over 90% is satisfied with the use of the
videocommunication. However throughout the whole period of use, clients
reported complaints about the technology involved, especially in the first year. The
complexity of use and the instability of the video communication were the main
complaints. In nearly 100 of a total of 760 h a combined audio and video contact
could not be arranged due to technical problems. To 13% of the participants these
technical problems were a sufficient reason to stop participation in the project.

The total number of participants at the end of the project did not reach the target
set at the start. This is due to the organizational changes that were made during the
project. A change in technology provider had to be accommodated at the

beginning of the project. Also the process of spontaneous marketing (clients acting as advocates of the videocommunication to their relatives) started slowly. The project started off by the special department of tele-services. In regular communication to care workers and clients only occasional communication on the progress of the videocommunication could be made.

During the project several initiatives were started to develop new applications. Examples are contact with general physician using the videocommunication and a memory support application. In addition, initiatives were taken to attract clients of other care organizations to participate in the project. Clients indicate that they are interested in the use of these newly developed applications.

The monitor activities delivered useful insight in the development of the project. The data gathered were used to guide the implementation activities. At the end of the monitoring period the data were also analyzed with respect to user satisfaction and effects at the user level. In part a comparison could be made between data gathered at the start of their participation and at the end of the project. A total of 85 clients completed both questionnaires. The tests showed that clients were very satisfied with the applications of the videocommunication. They showed a limited potential to actually pay for this kind of service. Over 65% of participants indicated that they are willing to pay less that 15 Euro a month, and only 5% indicated that they are willing to pay about 20–25 Euro. These amounts are insufficient to cover all the direct costs of this service. In judging this result it was noted that on the one hand it was highly unusual to pay for care services in The Netherlands and that this service was experimentally introduced as an extra service.

The perception of (personal) safety was monitored as well. The results showed a stabilization of the situation in most clients whereas in approximately one third an increase in unsafety was noted. These results were measured with a questionnaire in which items were included towards feelings of safety to live in their own apartment, the need of support to continue independent living. On the other hand the measurements of loneliness expressed at the individual level indicated that approximately 50% indicated a reduction of the sense of loneliness both at the social and at the emotional level (Fig. 6).

Measurements performed at the group level indicated that both at the social level and the emotional level of loneliness a significant reduction was noted. This result was obtained over a total period of 2 years with 85 clients. It gives a clear insight in the potential effects of the application of the videocommunication.

At the end of the project the care organization has taken the initiative to continue and expand the service.

4 Internal Influences on Development and Outcome

The project started as an initiative of the care organization department of "Telezorg" in close cooperation with the "technology in care" research department of Zuyd University. In cooperation with different companies the technical infrastructure was

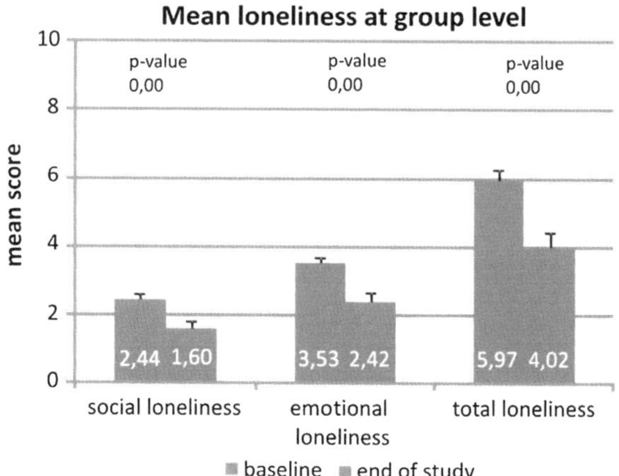

Fig. 6 Mean score social and emotional loneliness measured at the group level

organized. Also the initial applications were organized. The members of the care organization department were involved in identifying potential users and introduce them into the services. The team of Zuyd University was involved in the monitoring of the ongoing process by gathering data of use and interviewing the user at regular time intervals. Together with the care organization project leader, they were also involved in the research directed towards the identification of new applications for the videocommunication. The first example of a new application introduced during the project is the GMGA service. The role of the technology provider was to deliver and install the technology at the client's residence. During the project they implemented a revised version of the user interface. The call center used in this project, responsible for the direct contact with the clients was placed at Zuidzorg. They also registered data on the use of the service at the clients in case of the GMGA service.

The project described here was preceded by a small scale pilot initiated by the care organization. This was set up as a technology demonstration project. Upon completion of this project it became necessary, due to economical reasons, to attract a different technology provider. The selection of the technology provider also opened the opportunity to involve Zuidzorg in the project. They already had experience with the delivery of services to clients using a the videocommunication infrastructure.

No further changes in the organization of the project were undertaken.

5 External Influences on Development and Outcome

The delivery of care to people living independently in their own home is structured by law. Service delivery by homecare organizations is paid for by the law called AWBZ [3]. A selection process is used to identify the persons to whom this kind of service can be delivered. The homecare organization is paid for the delivery of this service. The technology involved is paid by a temporary experimental arrangement. Only a limited number of care organizations may use this source.

This situation is introduced by the fact that the government is reorganizing the structure of Dutch healthcare. It is the intention that the delivery of homecare will become the responsibility of local government. The legislative structure will gradually change into that direction. This change is introduced due to demographic and economic factors. This introduces for homecare organizations the need to develop new approaches to deliver their services to clients. The process of reorganization of healthcare is a complicated and time consuming process; at the national and regional level many parties are involved. It does not have a steady course. For the project this results in a complicated external environment. For project management this leads to the constant need to interact with an increasing number of organizations to keep the project on tract.

To obtain commitment of already existing clients and if possible to attract new clients the communication with care personnel outside the Telezorg department had to be intensified. Especially the use of technology as part of care delivery is a unfamiliar approach. Thus the communication with care workers about aims and approaches had to be intensified.

The technology provider received regular input with regard to the experiences of use. Especially the user interface appeared to be too complicated and had to be redesigned.

6 User Aspects

6.1 Introduction of Care Providers in the Videocommunication

The use of the videocommunication is a new approach of the care organization to deliver their services to the clients. As it is documented through research, care workers of the participating care organization (as well as others) are reluctant to use technology as part of care delivery [4]. This implied that a careful communication plan has to be organized towards these care workers to get them involved in the project as well. In company communication resources like newsletters, bulletin boards, explanatory presentations, and a organized partly in cooperation with regional patient organizations. Also to this group the above communication instruments are used.

During the project other care organizations are informed about the developments in this project. Up to this stage this has not led to an actual participation in the project. However at the time continuation is arranged, conditions are set to enable their participation as well.

6.2 Response of Users

User related aspects were intensively monitored during the project. At the start and at regular intervals thereafter users are interviewed on their experiences with the

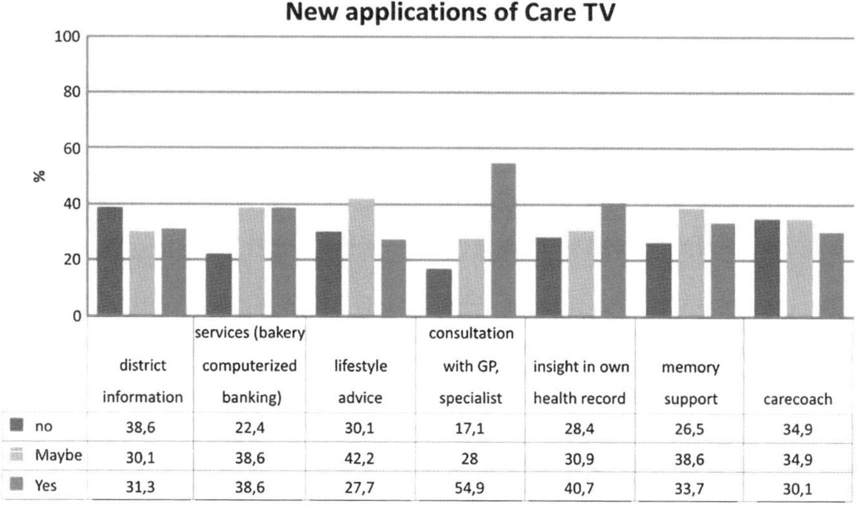

	district information	services (bakery computerized banking)	lifestyle advice	consultation with GP, specialist	insight in own health record	memory support	carecoach
no	38,6	22,4	30,1	17,1	28,4	26,5	34,9
Maybe	30,1	38,6	42,2	28	30,9	38,6	34,9
Yes	31,3	38,6	27,7	54,9	40,7	33,7	30,1

Fig. 7 Need for new applications expressed by users

project. The reactions received by the users were directed towards the use of the technology and the use of individual applications. In the beginning many complaints were received on the user interface. Controlling was integrated with the control of the TV set itself. After redesigning this interface users became more positive in their reactions. The use of their own TV set was seen as a positive feature of this service.

The service "Mantelzorgcontact" or contact with family members living elsewhere using he videocommunication was a service that in general is highly appreciated. However the technical conditions to set up the connection was considered far too complicated. From the first monitor report this has been communicated with the supplier of the technology. However due to technical and economical reasons this situation has not been improved yet. The continuation of this situation can be considered as a serious threat to the exploitation of the videocommunication.

During the monitor interviews respondents also reacted on the different applications supported by The videocommunication. The information service called "wegwijzer", giving access to regional information, was used seldom. This is partly due to the interaction as a response to questions by clients, and partly due to the fact that the videocommunication is not considered by the users as a source of this kind of information.

The responses to the GMGA service are in general positive. Users react very positive to the kind of support given (social contact, medication support) and to the quality of the service that is given.

On several occasions users also have given valuable input to the development of new services (see Fig. 7).

As can be seen from these data the development of the use of the videocommunication, in communication with the general physician, is most wanted by these users. Yet also a need for the use of this communication infrastructure in a non-care domain can be noted.

Being asked to their willingness to pay for these services most of the clients responded in a reserved way.

7 General Aspects

7.1 Outcome

As indicated with the data presented in Fig. 6 the use of the videocommunication renders an effect on the experienced loneliness by the user. Both the social and the emotional loneliness was affected in a positive way. At the level of safety no significant improvement could be noted in the comparison between before and after the use of the videocommunication. As a consequence of the experimental setup no comparison could be made with clients that are non-users of the videocommunication.

At the level of quality of labor the project has rendered only marginal effects up to now. The limited number of personnel involved and the limited number of applications are the primary cause. However, at the moment new applications are introduced and the use of the videocommunication is not only directed towards users but will become a regular tool of the care worker, it will also generate effects at the level of quality of labor. In this way care workers may become able to be connected to their clients in a more efficient way since they do not have to travel to the clients house.

7.2 Dissemination Strategy

The project has been started as an initiative of the care organization. Its main emphasis was directed towards both the identification of new services and towards the development of an innovative way of the delivery of services to the clients. The dissemination strategy chosen is a reflection of this. All existing clients will be contacted to stimulate them to use the videocommunication. Once the applications are well defined it will become possible to use them on other technical platforms enabling video communication as well. By that time it may very well be possible to join other service suppliers and combine efforts. The care organization is willing to use that strategy as well. To enable it, contacts are made with other care organizations active in the region as well as the health insurance board, service organizations in the living and welfare domain and local municipalities. Following these lines it must become possible to set up an arrangement in which the videocommunication becomes part of a social information and communication infrastructure. In the mean time the care organization will have to continue with the development of new applications as part of the telecare services.

8 Conclusion

In conclusion, the development of the videocommunication as a tool for communication between care organization and the client has been brought forward by this project. First effects at the client level are positive. Attempts to identify and organize new services are promising but require a good cooperation with several organizations in the region. Implementation of the applications into regular practice can now be undertaken.

References

1. Demiris G, Hensel BK. Technologies for an aging society; a systematic review of "smart home" applications Yearb. Med Inform. 2008; 33–40.
2. Willems ChG, Heide van der L, Spreeuwenberg MD. ZorgTV bij Proteion Monitor van gebruik tussen 2008 en 2010, Zuyd University.
3. AWBZ department of welfare, health and sports. healthcare in the Netherlands; The Hague Netherlands downloaded 24 August 2010 from http://www.minvws.nl/en/folders/cz/2005/health-insurance-system/default.asp.
4. Claus E. ICT in de Thuiszorg. Wetenschappelijk onderzoek naar de be factoren met betrekking tot de acceptatie van ICT door thuiszorgmedewerkers. Maastricht University, faculty of health, medicine and life sciences. 2007.

Establishing an Infrastructure for Telecare: Combining the Socio-Technical and the Clinical

Giovanni Rinaldi, Mike Martin and Antonio Gaddi

Abstract ICTs offer great opportunities for delivering telemedicine and social care in a number of domains including services for the elderly. This area of application, however, presents many challenges at many different levels. The purpose of this chapter is to describe an approach followed, and explore some lessons learned in Bologna (Italy). The stated objective of these developments was to maintain independent living, in their own homes, by elderly people for as long as possible and as cost effectively as possible. Thus the approach was an attempt to address the challenges both of the quality and the economics of care. Part of the background to the project was that, over the previous 10 years, more than three hundred elderly people had been involved in different home care projects in the Municipality. These initiatives started with traditional approaches to the integration of home care applications (telemedicine devices or software applications) using proprietary and ad hoc mechanisms and culminated in the development of the concept of a technical and organizational platform with the potential to overcome many of the problems of traditional e-Care applications and to exploit some of the new potentialities offered by network technologies such as eHealth and web 2.0 in health.

Keywords eHealth · Home care · Social care informatics · eCare · Socio-technical systems

G. Rinaldi (✉) · A. Gaddi
University of Bologna, Bologna, Italy
e-mail: giovanni.rinaldi@cup2000.it

M. Martin
University of Newcastle, Newcastle, UK

Commun Med Care Compunetics (2011) 3: 43–66
DOI: 10.1007/8754_2011_23
© Springer-Verlag Berlin Heidelberg 2011
Published Online: 8 May 2011

1 Introduction and Description of the Project

This chapter presents a multi-perspective view of what turned out to be a complex and emergent project. The attempt to discuss the work in terms of its clinical, political and technical backgrounds, its objectives and aspirations, the complex unfolding of events that took place and the learning and insights that were achieved, inevitably produces a narrative which spans a number of disciplinary perspectives. This underlines the multi-faceted nature of the task of introducing new forms of care through new channels and infrastructure.

The most inclusive expression of the requirement that the OLDES project addressed was "to promote and sustain the wellbeing of older people, at home and in the community, by providing an infrastructure and services capable of supporting the operation and governance of a dynamic and participative economy of care services". This chapter describes the reference architecture which creates a framework for the application of current ICT components to the challenging area of telecare of the elderly. The concept of telecare combines both telemedicine, in the form of monitoring and supervising clinical processes and "tele-accompany" which is concerned with the development and maintenance of social capital through contact and interaction. The concept of wellbeing that was being pursued did not allow these two aspects of care to be separated and treated independently. A consequence of this commitment was that the environment had to accommodate the operations of, and relationships between, different agencies in health, social care and the voluntary and private sectors facilitating their partnership and brokering their co-production, with their clients, of safe and satisfactory outcomes and life experiences. We had also to consider the high number of co-morbidities experienced by the elderly which demands caution and flexibility in the choice and delivery of health and social services. At a technological level, the project provided set-top boxes with broadband internet connection in the homes of the participants. In the clinical part of the experiments, data from monitoring devices such as blood pressure, heart rate and weight was connected wirelessly to the local home hub and transmitted from there to a clinical applications server for access by doctors. On the tele-accompany side, various content and communications resources were offered to the users including voice over IP call and conference services.

A technologically advanced home care environment implies a highly distributed technical and organisational network, composed of heterogeneous and autonomous nodes involved in supporting the elderly through the delivery or orchestration service. The service platform is designed to support the dynamic introduction of new services and new configurations, in response to evolving need, technical opportunities and financial conditions. The elderly are themselves actors in the network not only as recipients but as the providers of elements of care and mutual support. This approach implies a concept of federation rather than the more usual one of vertically oriented integration. An essential aspect of a care relationship is that the subject of care is known, appreciated, understood and respected by the providers of care. In network environments, the means of knowing and understanding "users" are embodied in technologies such as user profiling which detects, observes and analyses activities in the system. One of the significant issues to be addressed in the deployment of technologies for tele-care is how mechanisms of governance can be incorporated into the environment to ensure that technologies such as these remain ethical and acceptable under the consent of the user and are not interpreted simply as observation or even surveillance. These issues of governability have not been considered as particularly significant in the general development of web services and technologies and this represents a major issue in their deployment in the caring and developmental public service arena.

1.1 The Previous e-Care Projects

The project implemented in Bologna co-funded by the EU under the Ambient Assisted Living theme called OLDES [1] had the main scope to overcome the shortcomings of previous homecare projects [2]. They had the followings goals [3].

- To connect the stakeholders in social and health care processes: citizens and their families, General Practitioners, specialists, nurses, social assistants, and Health Trusts (public, private and non-profit);
- To integrate the information needed during the treatment, to provide more complete and better co-ordinated care using ICT solutions;
- To obtain a real co-ordination of health and social services through an effective and integrated network of information, transaction communication services;
- To collect citizens' health information through the network;
- To connect citizens to information on their own health by giving them an easy way to access the network and its content services.

The predominant target subjects for home care projects are older people living alone with or without chronic diseases. Other projects have been directed at people with disabilities or families with children having chronic health or social problems. The home care service for the elderly in Bologna started in 2006 at first as a tele-accompany service delivered from a contact centre. Its aim was to provide social and health services for elderly people living alone. Building on this foundation different targeted projects were implemented using monitoring devices for, for example, cardiopathic disease with over 300 elderly people with different degrees of disease being connected to the services. Funding from the EC VII Framework Programme provided an opportunity to build on and improve these interventions by developing and deploying an electronic service platform and the organisational structures and relationships needed to manage it.

1.2 The New Approach

An integrated system for the care of older people must include a number of agencies and organisations, such as Local Health Organisations, care centres, municipality social services and volunteer associations. It also involves the co-operation of a number of different individual actors such as social care assistants, health professionals, elderly people themselves and their friends and relatives. A technologically advanced e-Care environment which responds to and accommodates this heterogeneity has to deliver a highly distributed, collaborative network, composed of autonomous and semi-autonomous nodes each of which is involved in different aspects of delivering support and care and wellbeing.

We would like to stress the multi-dimensional nature of this notion of wellbeing [4]. It includes the concepts of social, human and cultural capital all of which are subject to change as the ageing process proceeds. The notion of community in our statement of requirement is also important. We are not only concerned with sustaining older people's ability to live safely and comfortably at home but also stress the links to social, human and cultural capital that "community" implies in both the physical and the virtual domains. Being at home and belonging to a community are not necessarily the same. Further, the term "home" implies intimacy, companionship and privacy. When these attributes are transferred to the necessarily institutional and legally bounded setting of public services, health and social care, they must be instrumentalised in terms of consents and ethical approvals. When attempts are made to virtualise them and to substitute alternative channels, modalities and media, then the process of offer, adoption and appropriation of new or transformed service by users and by carers must be appropriately facilitated if the process is not to be interpreted as a withdrawal rather than an offer of care. The term "infrastructure" is also significant in that it implies that users, both as practitioners and clients or as institutions and agencies, shape the patterns of use in response to their changing needs and priorities rather than have designers and implementers capture and fix their processes in an applications oriented way. This approach to providing infrastructural services, rather than structural applications, has two important consequences:

Firstly it accommodates the dynamism of the care ecology and the care economy. Ecology because there are many actors depending on each other, interacting and transacting in complex ways over the infrastructure and in the real, face to face world. New actors arrive and others depart, resources and policies emerge and evolve and balances shift: only the concept of an ecology is rich enough to express these patterns. Economy because there are hard limits on capacities and resources; optimisation and rationing are realities that must be faced while costs and demand are managed. Finally, health and social care operate in a public sector, and political economy. This includes processes of service planning, commissioning and performance assessment.

Secondly, the dynamism of the environment places a particular requirement on the way the mechanisms of governance are supported. The service oriented, infrastructural approach defines a clear horizontal boundary between those aspects of operation which are the responsibility of the infrastructural service provider and those that remain associated with the users, i.e., care service providers and their clients. These users, in the context of care service delivery, operate under strict codes of practice and of governance and these must be appropriately supported by the infrastructure.

1.3 The Description of the Technical Architecture

The requirements for privacy, consent and governance in the proposed environment implies a far finer grained and more directly and dynamically manageable set of mechanisms for access to, and use of, information that is generated within the system compared with the normal practice of commercial systems. To express these we have returned to some of the notions which were common in the traditional architecture of telecommunications systems. In the days of "Plain Old Telephone Service" the service access point (SAP) and the subscriber (User) Connection Point (UCP) provide two reference points in what is otherwise a conventional (hub and spoke/enterprise bus, etc.) systems approach. The purpose of these reference points is to provide clear partitioning between sets of functions which also correspond to the division of the rights and responsibilities of actors. Thus the SAP represents the boundary between subscriber equipment and the network while the UCP represents the single point in the infrastructure through which all the service data passes. It is at this point that the distinction and demarcation between traffic, that is to say content data and signalling data can be made explicit and acted upon. The former "belongs" to the users while the latter is needed by the service provider to deliver the requested service. Traffic is switched and routed without interpretation by the conventional communications system whereas signalling is passed to the management system for the purposes of control and billing. The reintroduction of this concept allows us to make certain issues of information governance and consent explicit at the highest level in the architecture. The concept of a UCP provides us with a means of defining, elaborating and locating functions which categorise service data according to purpose and consent. In summary, the conventional distributed information systems technologies make everything visible that is not explicitly encrypted. This is the reality of the Internet, as a public space, and within the enterprise solution, behind its defended boundary, as a single private space. The project for assisting the elderly can be neither public nor a single private space. The former is ungoverned and the latter does not respect the multi-agency nature of the care ecology/economy or the special status of care relationships. These issues become particularly important when we consider the use of technologies and techniques for profiling, customising and providing context sensitive support to users. Capabilities such as these, which are being offered as a means of facilitating and improving service, have

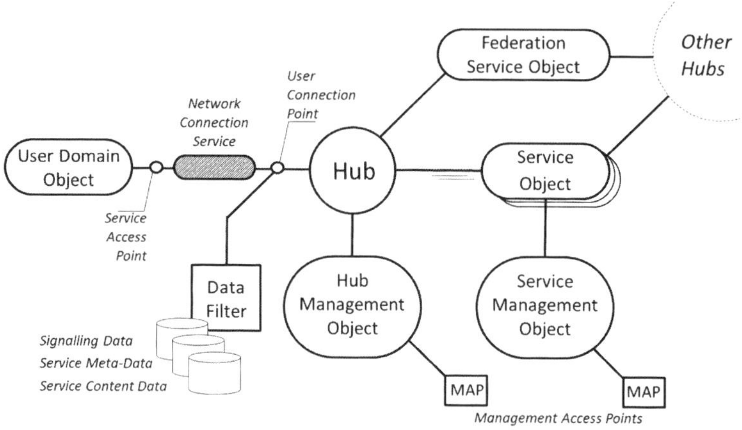

Fig. 1 OLDES architecture

been developed in the context of the Internet as a public space where publication is universal and there is no hindrance to access and use of data or the observation of data being used. If they are to be applied in the contexts of the health and social care of the elderly then they must be rendered governable and this governance must be open to inspection and participation to all the stake holders who have rights and responsibilities associated with it. Client information can only be accessed and used on the basis of consent and ethical principles. Sometimes that consent is implicit in the use of the service, on other occasions it might be regarded as traffic which can only be delivered but not interpreted by the service infrastructure.

1.4 The OLDES System Architecture

The highest level of abstraction and representation of the OLDES architecture (see Fig. 1) is centred on the Hub object. The Hub object contains three service sub components:

- The Portal-object which has the purpose of supporting the publication and syndication mechanisms required to support catalogues and directories of offers and availabilities in the partnership.
- The Switch-object which is concerned with the routing, ordering and co-ordination of messages, transactions and channels according to service processes and workflows.
- The Index-object which represents the capability and consent table defining which services (and users) can invoke which other services and service components in what contexts.

These objects are simply an abstract way of describing what is now considered the conventional functionality of middleware, i.e., of talking about the functionality which is currently implemented in the offers of the systems integrators.

The Hub object has connections to two classes of external functionality, User domain objects and Service objects:

The Hub object has connections to two classes of external functionality, User domain objects and Service objects:

A User Domain Object is connected to the hub by a standard network service such as WiFi or xDSL. The user domain object is composed of all the functions that are associated with the domestic equipment in the house of the elderly user but it should be noted that there could be several versions of this including fully functional PCs and client systems. The initial work of the project was based on the following sub-components of the User Domain Object.

- Set top box.
- Television with a remote control, microphone and SAP to the network.
- A set of clinical devices, fixed and portable sensors networked to the Set top box.

The connection of the User Object to the Hub is also shared by the Data Filter Object which is capable of monitoring all traffic and classifying it into three categories:

1. *Service signalling data* which is used to control the service process. This is recorded in the service network monitoring log where it may be accessed and used by management functions.
2. *Service meta* data which is descriptor data about the type of message/transmission which is taking place. It provides information about the type of content and the roles and contexts which the service session involves. This is also logged and provides an important input into the governance of practice and, through aggregation, to the planning and commissioning processes.
3. *Service content data* which is only logged or relayed to functions other than the addressed service end-points if there is a specific consent tag identifying the additional access rights and policies.

The Hub also has service objects connected to it. There are three sub-classes of service object and all of these inherit the basic capabilities of a service object in that their functions appear in the catalogues which define which other systems objects (service or user) that can access them and the uses that they can make of their data. There are several sub-types of Service Management Object. A Hub management object connects to a hub itself and also to the data filter object and controls its configuration and operation. Other services, accessing and using logged/monitored data do so through the access service provided by the Hub Management (service) Object. Service Management objects can also be associated with a service object where they are concerned with the configuration and the maintenance of quality of the service. Each service management object also has a Management Access Point to provide the external interface to its functions.

There are two sub-classes of service providing object. The first is associated with a "local" service, i.e., a service provided by an entity which is part of the partnership associated with the hub. Note that service objects may deliver service to more than one hub, e.g., National services. The concept of the architecture presented so far provides for multiple services to be offered independently. Services, however, interact at the technical, semantic and pragmatic levels. There are always constraints on the order and the combination of things that can be done in a multi-service environment due to interdependencies, side effects and capacities. It is the purpose of the P, S and I objects in the hub to provide appropriate supportive co-ordination and we refer to this as service logic. The principal mechanism for achieving this is the support of context sensitive browsing, navigation, selection and control dialogues with the user.

The federation service object is a special case of a third party service provider which allows for the federation of the OLDES environment. The sub-services provided by the federation service provider are concerned with hub to hub interactions, specifically:

P–P interworking services where elements of content publications and catalogues can be accessed and used remotely to support inter partnership service use and provision.

S–S interworking services where processes, transactions and workflows can be co-ordinated across partnership borders.

I–I interworking service which support identity and relationship management across boundaries.

Functionally, a federation service is similar to a hub but having hubs instead of applications as its "spokes". The difference is in the nature and participation in the governance. The emergence of federation services such as these to address the problems which are referred to in the language of enterprise solutions as "interworking" and offers an alternative to point to point adapters. The OLDES project did not be develop such services within its work plan but, they are essential to the development of the strategic vision of trajectories and convergence paths for the OLDES environment is to be sustainable and to be able to respond to the organisational as well as technical challenges of scaling the approach to regional and national levels.

1.5 The Services Implemented

The initial platform included a set of information and entertainment channels with live social networks animated by volunteers. A major challenge of the approach was the engagement of the wide range of not-for-profit agencies and volunteers' organisations who have an interest in populating these channels, the provision of appropriate and sustainable business cases and the provision of appropriate governance and diversity. In developing these channels, OLDES took social and cultural capital into account as well as considering the economic aspects of sustainability models. It was clear that the voluntary and not-for-profit sector had a potentially significant role and interest in the possibilities being created and efforts were made to engage these sectors in the shaping of the initial experiments and pilots. Tools were developed for signalling the uptake of channels and content to publishers and broadcasters as part of the service brokerage approach. The patterns of use of content on an individual level also provided potentially valuable data about changes and trends in the wellbeing of users which was supported by extensive classification and categorisation of content type supporting user profiling.

In the case of specific clinical monitoring of cardiovascular disease implementations of sphygmomanometer, weight scale, oximeter and single lead ECG devices for the detection of arrhythmias have been initially trialled. Data from these units is sent to a unit attached to the hub for record, analysis and decision making. A patient accessible space was also provided enabling them to perform activities such as completing questionnaires about their social state or chronic disease, make observations or to record a personal audio diary to provide information about their personal condition.

2 Development of the Project

At the outset of the project, the model of the relationship between service provision and service use was based on a clear tradition of public provision of welfare and care and of collective representation as the basis for participation. The project plan, however, called for participative design and there was a strong attempt from some members within the consortium to extend this to a co-productive approach in which demarcated provider—user relationships were broken down and a much more equal relationship and distribution of control was delivered. This represented a challenge to both practitioners and managers in their traditional relationships.

Meanwhile, considerable effort was devoted to the creation and delivery of engagement activities in which needs, wants and possibilities were explored with a wide range of actors, including many older people themselves, who had an interest or stake in the network.

2.1 The Evaluation of the Capability of the Elderly in the Use of Technology

The engagement with the elderly people in the focus group work was a feature of all stages of the development work, producing a better understanding of general and specific needs, preferences and capabilities. The first step in this process involved the administration of specific questionnaires. The method used is comparable with the results from another setting (laboratory population of Massa Lombarda near Bologna) [5, 6]. In this context we met 84 elderly people (mean age: 78 ± 6 years old, M:W = 1:1.2), grouped in ten associations or parishes. The interview was composed of 70 items and took approximately 15 min to complete. This process was conducted through interview in some cases and by the respondent alone in others. It consisted of four parts.

The first part, besides registry data, included a number of questions which explored the social network of the respondent including familial composition, frequency of contacts with relatives, capability of walking autonomously, means of transport usually used, cultural activities and level of education. The state of health of the subject was also investigated through questions about recent admissions to hospital, consultations with a general practitioner or specialist and eyesight, hearing and dental problems. A self-evaluation of health was also requested expressed in a scale from 1 to 5 (corresponding to "poor "and "excellent" respectively).

The second part was specifically dedicated to the use of technology enquiring about which tools were used in everyday life from a list of ten items including whether the subject could use a cell phone or a computer, whether they listen to the radio and/or watch TV and whether someone else in their family was capable of using technology.

The third part was about psycho–physical state including questions about what the respondents did when they felt lonely, whether they were ever depressed while at home and what they did in such cases, whether they regularly measure their blood pressure and whether or not they are able to do so on their own.

The fourth part was about ICT in medicine. The questionnaire included four questions about interest in ICT tools: (1) interest in an instrument to put people in contact with medical staff (2) interest in an instrument to measure some vital signs (3) interest in an instrument to communicate vital signs to medical staff (4) interest in having such an instrument with remote control.

The major aims of our analysis were: (1) to determine the level of knowledge elderly people have of ICT medical tools (2) to assess the interest in ICT (3) to look for factors which could influence attitude towards ICT.

Analysis of data must be cautious, due to the limited number of cases and the large number of factors which can influence results. However, this preliminary evaluation gave useful indications about further investigation. First of all, our data suggests that knowledge of ICT tools was quite poor among our group. This is not surprising, considering that systematic literature review shows that only very few sources of information "deal with presenting and customising health information for elderly and disabled people" [7]. However, results are in some way more encouraging regarding interest in ICT, even if considerable differences were present in our group. In order to suggest possible explanations for this variation, we looked for factors which could possibly influence their attitude towards ICT. We considered the impact that their state of health could have on an interest in ICT, because most users of telemedicine tools are suffering from complex, long term conditions. In our analysis, however, no significant correlation was found between health and interest in ICT.

It is not easy to evaluate the state of health of a person and the questionnaire contained several questions which investigated this area. In our analysis we used self evaluation of the state of health to perform a correlation with interest in ICT. Results of our analysis show that our group was composed of elderly people who are generally in good health. Due to the fact that the interviews were conducted in public places like clubs and parishes, this was not surprising and our data probably did not represent the general elderly population. An obvious reason which could influence the attitude of elderly people towards ICT is their capability of using technological tools in general. People who are not used to them could find it difficult to use ICT tools, and this could prevent them from even trying. That is why we dedicated an entire part of the questionnaire, consisting of seven items, to the use of technology. In general, the surveyed people had fairly good techno-logical skills, and there is a significant correlation between these skills and interest in ICT. This seemed to corroborate our initial hypothesis that familiarity with technology is the key factor in attitude towards ICT tools. An interesting and possibly counter—intuitive result of our analysis was that people who tend to go out more are also more interested in ICT, while people who find it difficult to move are often considered a primary target of ICT. Possible explanations of this data could be: (1) the fact that people who have more outside activities are more familiar with technological tools (2) people who have an outgoing personality tend to be more open towards new means of communication.

The preliminary study indicated that our selected cohort of quasi-healthy elderly people in Bologna had relatively little knowledge about ICT, but they were quite interested in ICT tools and their potential applications for health. Analysis of interest in ICT and several other variables (age, gender, level of education, state of health and isolation) do not show any significant correlation. These data seem to suggest that interest in ICT could be linked to a number of factors, including behavioural, cognitive and psychological ones, sometimes difficult to evaluate and not intuitive. Even if at the moment there is only a limited number of studies about this subject in the literature, our results were consistent with those of Williams et al. [8]. Further investigation is required to determine people's interest in ICT tools and therefore their impact on everyday medical practice and how this is changing with succeeding cohorts. The definition of a standard questionnaire would be very useful in order to make the results of different centres comparable and to gather large amounts of data. It seems necessary, for every kind of ICT tool, to consider the expectations and needs of the primary target this technology is aimed at. An effort should be made to analyse and empirically evaluate its acceptability and desirability among patients in different environments, with regard to several aspects (not only physical and cognitive, but also social, psy-chological, and so on, in order to have a global evaluation of potential users of ICT). This effort would contribute to giving e-health and telemedicine practice some solid and evidence-based support. The use of ICT *in corpore vili*, in other words, uses in which patients, especially elderly ones, are treated as passive actors in the process of getting, transmitting and elaborating medical information should not be considered acceptable.

From the clinical point of view one of the expectations regarding the telemonitoring of patients (e.g., patients with heart failure, or in chronic pain, or with diabetes) at home is to improve outcomes [9]. The detection of such improvements may be through the measurement of surrogate endpoints, for example the presence of oedema, heart rate and blood pressure levels, or the intensity of pain or blood sugar. Alternatively improvements may be measured by relevant outcomes (e.g., mortality, the occurrence of nonfatal new events or hospitalisations.) These goals must be considered and evaluated in the wider psychological and social context. Outcomes, however, measured, depend greatly on the ability of the elderly patient to use the telemedicine systems and that their reliable and accurate uses become part of the patients' daily lives. Achieving such a state of affairs through long term studies to test the feasibility, efficacy and efficiency presents many practical and ethical challenges. If the studies are not compatible with the lifestyles and personalities of the subjects, they can lead to confounding results but issues of lifestyle change and conformance to treatment are not separate and distinct issues; they are embedded in the care processes and relationships themselves.

This determines the clinical expectations in this area and places requirements of the systems that are supporting both clinical research and care to allow the real time verification of the results and the quality of life, both on the surrogate end points, and on outcomes; and the adjustment of the system (devices, software, training of users, system etc.) in real time.

3 Outcome of The Project

The benefit that is delivered through the introduction of ICT into healthcare (especially in the care of the elderly) is not simple to evaluate. There have been many projects concerned with telemedicine or involving technical instrumentation for assisting the elderly but most have been pilots engaged in the initial experimental and testing phase of introduction [10], [11]. In order to investigate some of the long term implications of these developments we have been exploring attitudes and understanding of this work based on the reactions and experience of 120 GPs in Bologna involved in caring for elderly people. The context of this investigation and analysis has been the three years of the advanced medical course for GPs which they have attended at Bologna University.

There is a strong consciousness among the GPs that the increase in life expectancy (in Italy from $m = 77, 2$ yrs $f = 82, 8$ in 2003 to $m = 78, 4, f = 83, 8$ in 2007) is producing a net increase of patients with complex long term conditions [12]. The trend is similar for several industrialised countries [13]. This generates a need for improved continuity of care which is now recognised as a key element in the National Healthcare System. The concept of continuous care in a long term condition involves constant monitoring to avoid transitions to acute episodes [14].

Delivering this type of care implies a mix of technological and ethical factors with organisational and legislative possesses. In general, the physicians have expressed concern about the complexity of this situation and the difficulty of integrating available resources and opportunities in the primary care setting.

The relationship of clinical care between the GP and the patient is the most persistent and continuous one. The concept of continuous complex care we are developing here implies a new and even stronger connection between them and with the other roles involved in the primary care processes and relationships. These include nurses, who perform home activities, specialists in the hospital setting who address specific health problems and social workers. All of these actors need to co-ordinate with the GP to manage the health and wellbeing of the patient as part of a continual process [15].

This model contrasts with the fragmentation of the care process in the traditional view which emphasises the concept of episodes of care. It also cuts across political issues governing the traditional differentiation of responsibility between care agencies which fails to provide a co-ordinated response to the patients complex and changing needs.

3.1 The Attempt to Improvement the Home Care for Elderly

In this section we will present a critical commentary on the unfolding story of the project in which we will attempt to highlight the key learning points which influenced the course of the project and the activities that it was undertaking and to underline its many faceted nature. There were two processes which were largely responsible for the detailed course of events in the project. Firstly, there were unforeseen disruptions which forced responses which were not fully foreseen in the original plan and, secondly, there were occasions where information was introduced from the outside or came to light within the project processes which provoked a reassessment and response.

We are focussing on these changes as the indicators of learning processes rather than as responses to breakdown in, or inadequacy of, the previous plan and the term "critical" here implies interpretive and evaluative rather than judgmental.

In order to re-establish the starting assumptions and priorities of the project, we will present an analysis of the Project Summary in which were summarised the main technical objectives to reach, for improving e-Care services in Bologna.

"The OLDES project will offer new technological solutions to improve the quality of life of older people. It aims at developing a very low cost and easy to use entertainment and health care platform designed to ease the lives of older people in their homes. In order to achieve this, new concepts developed in Information Technologies will be integrated and adapted. The platform will be based on a PC corresponding to Negroponte's paradigm of a € 100 device, giving the guarantee of an affordable system" [16].

It has been funded in a programme of technological research and its stance is one of technological determinism which asserts that, as long as the cost is acceptable, the adaptation and integration of technologies offers the solution to the presenting problem.

"OLDES will provide: *user entertainment* services, through easy-to-access thematic channels and special interest forums supported by animators; and *health care facilities* based on established Internet and telecare communication standards. The system will include wireless ambient and medical sensors linked via a contact centre to social services and health care providers" [16].

From the outset, the idea of an exclusively telemedicine system was rejected. This was based on previous experience of the strength and benefit of social support through the use of call centre mechanisms, however, the cost and scalability of the very personalised, one to one approach, was in question.

"OLDES will also cover the definition, implementation and evaluation of a Knowledge Management (KM) program, an advanced user profiling system that will enhance the communication between all the stakeholders of the system" [16].

The aspirations to include these sorts of technologies without acknowledging the ethical and social implications underlines the determinist frame in which the original proposal was written. The assumptions that there were no barriers to the deployment of a sufficient body of content and the collection of a critical mass of real user data to make the use of this technology feasible, all proved problematic.

"OLDES puts older people at the centre and makes their needs the main priority in all developments. This will be achieved through the use of modelling and animation tools to create scenarios designed to elicit responses from older people, their carers, and service providers" [16].

Here the emphasis is on the service network and environment.

So, the picture that emerges at the initiation of the project is of a number of groupings with very different stances and attitudes to the work to be undertaken. These can be summarised as follows:

The technical development perspective: we have an interesting new platform to work with and a concept of the system which is based on a home hub linking the TV, clinical devices, VoIP hand set and remote control to an ADSL link. A centralised service system will provide the content, communications and data collection services.

No special requirements for service management support is identified and all the services are assumed to be internal parts of a single system.

The Clinical Perspective: prior to the initiation of the project, the engagement of the clinical community has been at a Health Service level mediated by the Municipality and driven by the political sponsorship of the project. The reality on the ground soon reveals itself to be one of deep suspicion and scepticism.

Social Care perspective: no project resources were allocated to the Social Services units who were to be involved and the assumption of the Municipality was that they could order and control the required resources.

Municipality perspective: In their role as the provisioners and managers of service, the view of e-Care is business as usual. The collective representatives of the users will be informed about the system and their support in managing the rollout and use of the system will be won. There seems to have been an assumption that service content did not present a challenge and that it could be acquired or created without much difficulty.

We can summarize the technical outcome of the project through four phases. The main achievements of the first stage of work were:

1. The concept of a service architecture based on a (potential network of) brokerage hub(s) which connects user systems to a distributed set of local and remote service systems.
2. A layered service architecture making use of some traditional communications service systems concepts.
3. An approach to the issues of service management and governance to addresses the issues of consent and confidentiality which included the concept of provisioning and permissioning services to access and share data with each other as well as controlling the access of users and service providers to services.
4. An initial representation of and engagement of the main sections of the OLDES Network in the clinical, social care and public service commissioning domains.

The new conception of the home care environment represented a long term view. The next phase of the project was characterised by the growing awareness of the stability problems associated with the domestic platform. During this period, the idea of developing some user generated data on needs and preferences was introduced and the first round of focus group work involved real potential users. This directly achieved two things: firstly it maintained contact and engagement and secondly it did provide some insight for the priorities of the design of the system. It also had the indirect effect of establishing the three cornered approach and relationship between project members, the Voluntary organisations and the end users rather than the assumed previous configuration in which the project spoke to the Voluntary sector representatives and they spoke to their members.

These interactions were developed further into the concept of the "OLDES Lab". These are occasions at which e-Care users or potential users are brought together around some issue of interest or value for discussions, presentations and exercises. These activities generate content and relationships which can be further deployed and developed through network interactions.

The last phase of deployment involved the installation of systems in the home environments and the delivery of network nurturing activities in which animators promote activity by calling users and new content is introduced and promoted on the network. The importance of a smooth and simple installation process has been underlined in this process and it is clear that it cannot be treated as simply a technical task but must include an introduction and facilitation process which is sensitive to the needs of the user.

4 OLDES as Change and Development: Innovation Issues

The introduction of tele-medicine and tele-accompany services represents a significant transformation of care processes and enterprise and the creation, sustaining and governance of new capabilities and capacities. The leadership, vision and energy to make such changes a reality involve a sort of entrepreneurialist initiative. This, however, is an entrepreneurialism which operates in the public sector and Civil Society rather than in the market and the experience of the OLDES project raises important questions about the sources and the relationships between innovations in the technical, clinical and social domains.

4.1 Public Service Innovation

The visions of telecare we have been discussing imply innovation and initiative in the creation of new care enterprise. Traditionally, this is the role of the entrepreneur and the question arises, where do we look for the entrepreneurialism that will initiate new infrastructure and services such as envisaged by OLDES? For the purposes of this discussion we need a very broad and inclusive concept of "enterprise" so we define it as the organisation of resources in pursuit of a vision in the context of a set of norms and values. All of these factors may be dynamic and subject to externally and internally induced change. The success of an enterprise is judged in terms of:

1. Accumulation of a capital (symbolic or monetory).
2. Distribution of value (to members, clients, investors/commissioners and externals).
3. Sustainability/persistence.

We stress that we are not limiting ourselves to the usual domain of commercial enterprise but include social, cultural and political enterprise where the form of the organisation may be an association, a party, a club, an administration, a social enterprise or a non-profit company. (This is by no means an exhaustive list.) We further stress that the capital, investment, goods and dividends of enterprise can be based on human, social, cultural, political or spiritual value as well as financial value. Finally, entrepreneurship entails the leadership qualities to instigate the foundation and life of an enterprise. This takes different forms in the different domains we have identified: the clinical entrepreneurialism, for example, seeks to establish and maintain the skills, knowledge and specific capacity to deliver a certain type of clinical relationship or intervention while political entrepreneurialism seeks to establish and maintain an administration.

4.2 Operational and Change in Enterprise and Network Innovation

In operation, an enterprise exercises its organisation and resources in the execution of its plans and processes and evaluates the outcomes against its visions and mission. Sometimes, the enterprise reviews and adjusts its vision and mission and redesigns its plans and processes. The latter is a creative process of direction in the context of enterprise while the former are the process of management and delivery. On occasion, the revision(ing) process can be more profound; sense making is provoked in response to contradictions, ambiguities or discoveries and this may lead to a re-conceptualisation of the situation and context. This is working on the shared world view rather than in it. Sense making leads to changes in language and attitude which in turn results in new commitments to visions which could not have been articulated in the old concepts and language.

In cybernetic terms, the loop that moves from visions to plans, execution and evaluation is first order. It represents adaptive, goal directed behaviour which is accounted for in terms of learning, creativity and delivery within the bounds of a fixed conception of possibilities and values. The second loop, which places the first one in the context of sense making, re-conceptualisation or "languaging" and commitment is a second order cybernetic which corresponds to Gregory Bateson's deutero learning and we will equate to the concept of innovation [17].

In the light of this conception of enterprise, the entrepreneur is required to provide leadership in any or all of the areas of management and delivery, creative direction and innovation depending on the external and internal circumstances. There is a further requirement to facilitate the transitions and interfaces between these modes of activity and regards the network innovation proposed in this approach. It is based on a simple concept of the enterprise and its environment and says little about the relationships between the two or among enterprises. This lack can be remedied rather simply if we assume a commercial environment where the range of relationships between the elements of an economy are relatively simple and the system of value is uniform and universal. We have surveyed the mixed economy which is the OLDES environment which spans political, clinical and social as well as commercial domains and the overall OLDES vision of fully embedded infrastructure through which services to support the care and wellbeing of an ageing population are delivered and governed. It implies co-ordinated and mutually co-productive entrepreneurial innovation in several different sectors. It also implies a co-ordinated sequence of mutual adaptations which, in retrospect, are interpreted as path effects of the form "b was possible because a had been established" while in prospect, they represent strategic initiatives and responses. Finally, our theory of innovation implies that the process will involve changes of meaning and the creation of new language and values the details of which cannot be predicted.

5 External Influences on Development and Outcome

In this section we will consider the kinds of organisations, institutions and interests involved in e-Care service including the OLDES extension project. In doing so, we will again underline the mixed nature of the service economy and provide a basis for developing a theory of innovation and development against which the actual performance of the project and the outcomes it has produced can be assessed.

The care and support of the elderly involves a complex array of formal and informal services and relationships. From a clinical perspective, the logics of care which apply here include the full range of maintenance, remedial, preventative and palliative interventions. In the OLDES approach, the delivery of these interventions is situated in the community and in the home. The close combination of telemedicine with tele-accompany, social-networking and a potentially wide range of multi-media content based cultural and entertainment services has been a central feature of our approach. During the roll-out phase of the project, the importance of the balance between interaction mediated through the electronic means of the network and face to face events and interactions began to emerge, emphasising the principle that, in a development such as this, artificial boundaries on what is in scope or out of scope cannot be maintained and one of the most important criteria for success is that the network has taken on a life of its own rather than simply produced what was expected.

From an organisational perspective, we can partition the OLDES network into a number of domains which are differentiated by their respective interests and responsibilities.

5.1 The Clinical Domain

The traditional split of clinical service into the continuous and open relationship of primary care and the episodic and specialised care of hospital based, secondary care masks many of the realities of the care of the elderly. Ageing has been described as a complex, long term condition with only one prognosis and, even in the strict domain of clinical intervention, the range of agencies and practitioners, and the relationships between them, can be complex and dynamic [18]. One of the potential impacts of the introduction of telemedicine infrastructures and services is on the traditional concepts of ambulatory care, of the "in-patient" and the "out-patient" and of the division of responsibility and control of care among the patient, the GP and the specialist to say nothing of the relationship between clinical and social care. In relation to the question of the initiation of telehealth services and environments, we must question where the expected leadership (which we will equate to a form of entrepreneurialism) in the health service domain can or should come from: is it management led or practitioner led, will it be initiated in the primary or secondary care sectors, or, indeed, will telemedicine be a factor which will be seen as an external imposition on the health sector as a whole and, if so, is it to be resisted or accepted?

In particular the domain of the care of the elderly generates a strong require-ment for partnership and co-ordination between clinical and social care and within social care, the demarcation between formal services and the support at the informal, familial and community levels becomes blurred. An important aspect of these relationships it that they span significant boundaries between the apparatus of the State as the provider of public service, the Civil Society of the Voluntary Sector and Charities, and the market. Practical, working relationships which are effective in spanning these sectors tend to be based on trust rather than on formal structures and nurturing and promoting such trust is one of the most important aspects of the emergence of infrastructure.

5.2 Political Relationships: Municipality and Region

OLDES was initiated with very strong political sponsorship. The political sig-nificance of the ageing population as a constituency and the opportunity for Framework funding generated extremely strong political sponsorship. From this perspective, in the Emilia Romagna Region of Italy, many of the service resources for the care of the elderly are seen as aspects of the apparatus of the state in a context in which Welfare and Public Service are seen as significant responsibilities of public administration. Collective representation and action is also a significant aspect of this political milieu and, in the context of the ageing population this is reflected in the membership and active participation of voluntary associations and other organisations. In the early stages of the OLDES project, the concept of participation and user centeredness was seen from the standpoint of the Munici-pality, as a matter of official, collective rather than individual engagement. The broadening and deepening of this conception of engagement has been a significant feature of the learning processes of the project.

6 User Aspects

As we have indicated, there was a strong commitment to direct user engagement in participative design [19] and co-production in the OLDES project among what can appropriately be called the "social science" oriented members of the OLDES consortium who saw it as their responsibility to help and encourage partners to adopt what was for them a new and sometimes challenging approach [20].

In the early phase of the project, interactions with the voluntary organisations had proceeded as planned but reached a point where the perceived need was to "show them a real system". This, however, was problematic because of the hardware delays and it was in this period that the idea of developing some user generated data on needs and preferences was introduced. A first round of ques-tionnaire and focus group work was undertaken under the aegis of the selected

Social Centre and the Parish, and involving real potential users. This directly achieved two things: firstly it maintained contact and engagement and secondly it provided insight for the priorities of the design of the system. It also had the indirect effect of establishing the three-cornered approach and relationship between project members, the voluntary organisations and the end users rather than the assumed previous configuration in which the project spoke to the voluntary sector representatives and they spoke to their members.

Interactions with users continued and has been developed into the concept of the "Lab" events. These are occasions at which the users or potential users are brought together around some issue of interest or value for discussions, presentations and exercises. These activities generate content and relationships which can be further deployed and developed through network interactions.

These interactions with users intensified with the roll out of more systems.

The process of installation and introduction in the home required care in planning and skill in execution to ensure that it was a positive experience for the user which encouraged them to adopt and use the equipment. Informal evidence of user perceptions and reactions during this period were mixed. Some adopted and accepted the role of "pioneer" and were encouraged to see themselves as innovators within the project. Interestingly, the subjects in the clinical trials proved resilient and responsive in this respect. Others proved less resilient.

Evidence continues to accumulate about the need for active nurturing and development of the network and the user community which, perhaps, should not be interpreted as a problem but as an inevitable part of the investment in building and sustaining social and human capital.

7 General Aspects

The impact of the project on efficiency, quality of labour, quality of care and quality of life has not, at this early stage, been established. However, the need to provide tools and mechanisms for making these assessments and ensuring that the ongoing governance of the network and the services it is providing can be supported with real evidence has been addressed in the design of the system.

Instrumentation to collect data on network behaviours and traffic has been built into the design of the infrastructure and data, which is anonymous, can be aggregated and displayed in different ways to detect which resources are being used and which pattern levels of communication and interaction are being exercised.

7.1 Market and Private Provision of Care

The role of commercial supply of care services has not figured highly in the OLDES project, reflecting the political and market realities of Emilia Romagna.

However, any infrastructure oriented approach to the organisational and technical design of the environment must take into account that this is not a universal situation and that in many contexts, in which systems are based on the OLDES architectural approach, there may be high, even dominant private provision. Even within an environment where provision of service is a balance between the State and the Civil Society, the element of choice and of competition between suppliers in relation to clients is never completely absent, so, from the outset, it has been a recognised requirement on OLDES to support the delivery and governance of market like mechanisms and relationships.

7.2 *Infrastructure Provision and Service Brokerage*

While the concept of brokerage did not figure in the original proposal, the initial phase of the project produced a shared understanding of the significance of the role in a service environment and that many aspects of service brokerage were being exercised by members of the consortium in their day to day operations. The ability and willingness of certain actors in the network to provide brokerage and the acceptance of others to be brokered is an essential aspect of any service infrastructure and is critical to its governability. The application of these principles in the context of the deployment and adoption of new channels and media represents one of the greatest challenges in the creation of infrastructure and in service innovation.

8 Conclusions

The core of the experiences of the project can be summarized as follows:

- The processes of creating and deploying an infrastructure are not compatible with clinical trialling, it is essential to establish the environment technically, socially and organisationally before any attempt at clinical science, in the strict sense of the term, is undertaken. Only then is there the possibility of laboratory controlled conditions. However, from the outset, questions of clinical and social effectiveness have to be considered.
- The classification of problems as clinical or social itself becomes problematically multi-perspective, in the care of the elderly, leading to particular difficulty in the establishment of base lines and classifications for epidemiological work. Simple causal links between conditions, interventions, clinical outcomes and quality of life become difficult to observe and capture, even less measure with any precision and reliability.
- As indicated above, in the home environment the scope cannot be limited to the clinical but must include social (cultural, spiritual...) care, furthermore the

target of the project demands a continuity of assistance and not an approach based on episodic encounters.

- The engagement of the elderly and the design of user friendly devices and services through a serious engagement in participative design and trialling was one of the most important challenges of the project.
- The delivery of care in the home depends on the establishment of a complex network of service supply relationships of many different sorts and with significant elements of trust and dependency. It is not possible to legislate, design and manage these relationships into existence, they represent transformational change and the development of new trust and partnership.
- The sequence in which different aspects of a complex service system is introduced involves selection, prioritisation, and path effects in the context of a number of explicit and emergent constraints. In the face of this uncertainty and ambiguity, it has been essential to maintain the close engagement of the representatives of all members of the network in all aspects of governance and management decision making.

The nurturing of this network into existence and the creation of appropriate governance as well as management structures is at the heart of the problem of establishing this kind of innovation and development.

About the innovative processes (clinical, technical and social) the progress of the OLDES project has produced significant changes in the conception of, and attitude to, many aspects of care service provision among the members of the care networks involved. Had the extent to which such changes were necessary been clear at the outset, it is doubtful whether the project would have started at all. The areas of innovation which can be identified in the OLDES story include the recognition of the following:

- That, in the case of telemedicine, the relationship between clinical interventions which are designed, delivered and evaluated according to a well established practice of clinical science and the technical infrastructure and environment in such work is undertaken is a complex one. You cannot do experiments until you have at least the basis for an appropriate laboratory and in the case of telemedicine, this has social and organisational as well as technological aspects.
- Establishing a technical infrastructure for the delivery of an economy and ecology of services is complex and challenging. The conventional approaches of management and systems development are poorly adapted to dealing with the resulting ambiguity and uncertainty.

In the light of the results of the service implemented for the elderly we can reformulate the initial assumptions and this implies a new set of needs and questions. These include:

- Can a network of telecare services be initiated in isolation or must it be symbiotic with an outgrowth of established infrastructure and services? Will the vision only be achieved when "home automation" and the "Internet of objects" in which many domestic appliances will be networked become the norm? If this is the case, the technical, organisational and political questions of governance we have discussed at some length here, remain.

- At what point in the emergence of a telecare infrastructure can telemedicine services be introduced? Where can the clinical trial model be applied and when?
- What initiation and diffusion models are useful and appropriate?
- Where are the clinical entrepreneurs? Usually in specialism and not in service management/commissioning. Implications?
- How and when will a market for, and integration of, telecare devices, with accreditations and standards and how can it be encouraged when current conditions promote stand alone products?
- How are the concepts of harm and freedom, welfare and community, changing in a world of ambient information and communication and, in the face of this, what are the limitations/boundaries of systems of care?

References

1. OLDES project. www.oldes.eu.
2. Fitch CJ. Telemedicine to support the elderly in the UK. Health Inform J. 1999;5:128–35.
3. Rinaldi G, Tomba R, Lena C. La presa in carico elettronica del cittadino nel processo di assistenza: l'esperienza e-care nell'area metropolitana di Bologna. In: Salute e Società. E-Care e Salute. 2/2003: 93–114. Franco Angeli, Genova; 2003.
4. Reed J, Cook G, Childs S, McCormack B. A literature review to explore integrated care for older people. Int J Integr Care. serial on line Jan 14; 5. 2005.
5. Bove M, Carnevali L, Cicero AF, Grandi E, Gaddoni M, Noera G, Gaddi AV. Psychosocial factors and metabolic parameters: Is there any association in elderly people? The Massa Lombarda Project. Aging Ment Health. 2010;9:1–6.
6. Nascetti S, Linarello S, Scurti M, Grandi E, Gaddoni M, Noera G, Gaddi A. Assessment of the health status in the Massa Lombarda cohort: a preliminary description of the program evaluating cardio-cerebro-vascular disease risk factors and quality of life in an elderly population. Arch Gerontol Geriatr Suppl. 2004;9:309–14.
7. Marschollek M, Wolf KH, Effertz B, Haux R, Steinhagen-Thiessen E. ICT-based health information services for elderly people: past experiences, current trends, and future strategies. Med Inform Internet Med. 2007;32(4):251–61.
8. Williams TL, May CR, Esmail A. Limitations of patient satisfaction studies in telehealthcare: a systematic review of the literature. Telemed J E Health. 2001;7(4):293–316.
9. Naham ES, Blum K, Scharf B, Friedmann E, Thomas S, Jones D, Gottlieb SS. Exploration of patients' readiness for eHealth management program for chronic heart failure: a preliminary study. J Cardiov Nurs. 2008;23(6):472–3.
10. Barlow J, Singh D, Bayer S, Curry R. A systematic review of the benefits of home telecare for frail elderly people and those with long-term conditions. J Telemed Telecare. 2007;13(4):172–9.
11. Whitten P, Johannessen LK, Soerensen T, Gammon D, Mackert M. A systematic review of research methodology in telemedicine studies. J Telemed Telecare. 2007;13(5):230–5.
12. Minford M. The boundaries between health and social care for older people in developed economies. London: The Nuffield Trust; 2001.
13. European Commission. Confronting demographic change: a new solidarity between the generations. European Commission 94 Brussels. 2005.

14. Payne S, Kerr C, Hawker S, Hardey M, Powell J. The communication of information about older people between health and social care practitioners. Age Ageing Mar. 2002;31(2):107–17.
15. Magnusson L, Hanson E, Brito L, Berthold H, Chambers M, Daly T. Supporting family carers through the use of information and communication technology. Int J Nurs Stud. 2002;39(4):369–81.
16. OLDES: older people's e-services at home. Annex I description of work. FP6-2005-IST-62 IST-2005-2.6.2-AAL. Contract number 045282.
17. Gregory Bateson. Steps to an ecology of mind. University Press New edition, Chicago; 2000.
18. Mccoy H, Vila CK. Tech knowledge: introducing computers for cordinated care. Health Soc Work. 2002;27(1):71–4.
19. Suchman L, Schuler D, Namioka A. Participatory design: principles and practices. Lawrence Erlbaum Associates Inc, USA; 1993.
20. Hartswood M, Procter R, Slack R, Vob A, Buscher M, Rouncefield M, Rouchy P. Co-realization: towards a principled synthesis of ethnomethodology and participatory design. Scandinavian J Inform Syst. 2002;14(2):9–30.

Application of Teleophthalmology in Screening and Monitoring of Elderly Population in Rural Areas in Lithuania

A. Paunksnis, V. Barzdziukas, R. Gricius, D. Buteikiene, P. Treigys,
S. Kopsala, D. Imbrasiene, A. Maciulis, M. Paunksnis, L. Valius,
K. Andrijauskas and O. Tiihonen

Abstract A small regional telenetwork has been established in Lithuania and used
for piloting homecare and remote care health care service delivery models on
the grounds of the work of the Telemedicine Centre of the Lithuanian University
of Health Sciences (formerly Kaunas University of Medicine) and private initiative
of clinicians and researchers with the aim to promote bottom-up, self-sustainable
telemedicine development and to increase accessibility to, and quality of,
healthcare especially in rural or underserved areas. Stratelus, a small medical
company, together with several family clinics in the rural areas of Lithuania and
with support of the Family Medicine Centre of the Kaunas University of Medicine

A. Paunksnis (✉) · V. Barzdziukas · D. Buteikiene · A. Maciulis · M. Paunksnis
Stratelus JSC, Naugarduko 3, Vilnius, Lithuania
e-mail: alvydas@stratelus.com

S. Kopsala
Optomed OY, Hallituskatu 13-17D, Oulu, Finland
e-mail: Seppo.Kopsala@optomed.fi

P. Treigys
Vilnius University, Vilnius, Lithuania

L. Valius
Family Clinic of Lithuanian University of Health Sciences, Kaunas, Lithuania

O. Tiihonen
Remote Analysis OY, Konalantie 6-8B, 00370, Helsinki, Finland
e-mail: ossi.tiihonen@remoteanalysis.net

A. Paunksnis · V. Barzdziukas · R. Gricius · D. Buteikiene · D. Imbrasiene
Lithuanian University of Health Sciences, Kaunas, Lithuania

A. Maciulis
Kaunas University of Technology, Kaunas, Lithuania

K. Andrijauskas
Kaltinenai Primary Care Centre, Kaltinenai, Lithuania

Commun Med Care Compunetics (2011) 3: 67–87
DOI: 10.1007/8754_2011_27
© Springer-Verlag Berlin Heidelberg 2011
Published Online: 14 May 2011

started screening and monitoring of elderly population for diabetic retinopathy, aging macular degeneration, optic nerve head evaluation, and glaucoma in their homes and near-home locations, in a mobile telenetwork mode, bringing the access point to the patient. The project demonstrated innovation in terms of the methodology (telehomecare), organization (small bottom-up structure), and technology (high quality handheld fundus camera). The argument behind this project was to test the viability of homecare and remote care service delivery in a small/medium scale, bottom-up organisational setting. This is important for elderly population with limited mobility in rural or remote areas.

Keywords Telemedicine · Ophthalmology · Screening · Monitoring · Rural areas · Homecare · Telenetwork

Population groups included healthy people and patients clinical symptoms. Focus was on 3 clinical conditions at this stage—diabetic retinopathy, age-related macula degeneration and glaucoma.

Patient eye fundus images acquired while visiting them at home or seeing at near-home locations (virtually at home considering the distance) were sent by local family physicians/general practitioners to the competence center of Stratelus where they are being evaluated by tertiary level specialist physicians and evaluation results with clinical recommendations are sent back to the local family physicians. This project has improved accessibility to advanced diagnostics and timely healthcare for a number of rural elderly population who otherwise would often choose not, or could not to, travel to tertiary level healthcare providers for advanced diagnostics until late stage of symptoms. The overall outcome of the project is that initiation and delivery of small/medium telehomecare projects is possible, it can produce good clinical results, and they can be well received by all involved (patients, local physicians, tertiary level physicians), run on small budgets and have good chance to be self-sustainable in long-term.

1 Project Description

Access to health care is generally perceived as a right in many communities, especially in Europe. One of the priorities highlighted by the European Commission is ensuring that the results of biomedical research will ultimately reach the citizens. However, current demographic, economic, and social conditions are challenging effective and efficient delivery of health care services. Lithuania, as many other countries, has seen a combination of stress in public finance, ageing population, decrease of access to health care services in rural areas [1–6]. On the other hand, we have seen rapid growth of technologies, both imported and locally grown, and ICT boom. That prompts to explore possibilities of telemedicine [7–10].

The project "Application of Teleophthalmology in Screening and Monitoring of Elderly Population in Rural Areas in Lithuania" focused on using the telehomecare model in delivering services to patients in rural communities.

Telehomecare is a developing area of healthcare services that will provide significant benefits to the care providers their patients. Telehomecare is defined as "the use of communications and information technology to deliver health services and exchange health information to and from the home (or community) when distance separates the participants". Telehomecare in ophthalmology brings some real challenges, because in order to make correct ophthalmological diagnosis, a physician needs to evaluate relevant images which requires availability of a high quality equipment which up until recently was rather expensive [11–14]. Digital handheld equipment for ophthalmology was recently introduced to the market which helps to overcome some of these challenges. It can be used not only in general practitioner's office, but can be used for patients homecare as well.

In countries like Lithuania where large hospitals dominate the health services providers market seeing large centrally initiated projects is the norm. However, as primary care provision is continuously moving toward smaller physician offices and family clinics, smaller projects coming from local initiative are becoming increasingly important and they may have large impact for local communities. However, they need access to technologies, cooperation of various stakeholders local, primary care and tertiary level physicians), and some support and encouragement to stay motivated. To try address these issues and bring services closer to the patients, a small telenetwork has been established in Lithuania on the grounds of the work of the Telemedicine Centre of the of Lithuanian University of Health Sciences and private initiative of clinicians and researchers with the aim to promote bottom-up, self-sustainable telemedicine development and to increasing accessibility to, and quality of, healthcare especially in rural or underserved areas. Stratelus, a small company which is also the coordinator of the EU-supported Eurostars project, together with several family clinics in the rural areas of Lithuania and with support of the Family Medicine Centre of the of Lithuanian University of Health Sciences started screening and monitoring of elderly population for diabetic retinopathy, aging macular degeneration, and optic nerve head evaluation in remote family clinics and their homes, in a mobile telenetwork mode, bringing the access point to the patient's home. This is important for elderly population with limited mobility in rural areas.

Telehomecare has proven to be a good model for our project. In rural communities, the demand for tertiary level health care services is high, while patient and physician contact is still very personal and home visits are still often a form of health care services delivery. Telehomecare extended the existing primary care services to a higher specialist level. In terms of the end-user, the project was a combination of homecare and "near-homecare" i.e., provision of care within the community, at a primary care clinic at a proximity so close to home (within 10 min travel time) as compared with the tertiary healthcare centre, that it could virtually be considered homecare.

2 Development of the Project

2.1 Arguments for Initiating the Project

The overall argument for initiating this project was to test the viability of homecare and remote care service delivery in a small/medium scale, bottom-up organisational setting. All the ophthalmologists participating in the project have long experience working in the tertiary level healthcare institutions such as the Eye Clinic of the Lithuanian University of Health Sciences (formerly Kaunas University of Medicine) Hospital and currently hold their main clinical appointment there. Their observation was that patients who don't need tertiary level care are often referred to the tertiary level. Another group of patient is those who come to the tertiary level at a very late stage. As most of the participating ophthalmologists have also been active in the activities of the Telemedicine Centre of the Lithuanian University of Health Sciences, an initiative developed to use the expertise in developing a regional telenetwork and offering services closer to the patients, at home or near home (at local primary care clinics). On the other hand, for Stratelus, as a company, this offered an opportunity for offering new services as well (although financial gains were not a factor as services were generally provided at cost and with some sponsors' help). For patients though, the services offered economic benefits as discussed in Sect. 5.1.

2.2 Clinical Goals and Expectations

Our aim was to establish and develop telenetwork for homecare and remote care in ophthalmology in selected locations in Lithuania and test the viability of bringing the services and diagnostics closer and faster to the patients via telehomecare.

Objective 1. To provide infrastructure (mobile digital medical diagnostic systems—fundus camera and camera for anterior segment).
Objective 2. To train the primary care medical personnel on new telemedicine diagnostic equipment and technologies.
Objective 3. To perform preventive eye disease screenings and early diagnostics.
Objective 4. To perform monitoring of chronic diseases seeking minimization of complications.

This chapter presents the results of 4 establishments of teleophthalmological services in 4 rural or remote areas of Lithuania (Vilkaviskis, Karmelava, Kaltinenai, Klaipeda).

2.3 Innovative Elements

There were 3 kinds of innovative elements in the context of this project—methodological, organisational, and technological. In terms of the methodology of healthcare services delivery via telemedicine or telehomecare, although these methods have been implemented in some specific areas (emergencies; military), it has not become part of routine delivery in Lithuania yet, so the mode itself was an innovative element to the end-users. Organisationally, an innovative element was that this project emerged as a small project driven by bottom-up initiative. Technologically, and in the context of the clinical specialty (ophthalmology), the use of a handheld digital fundus camera for patient examination and data acquisition was an enabling factor to carry out this project.

3 Outcome of the Project

The project reached the aim as the viability of bringing the services and diagnostics via telehomecare was shown to be possible, and services were made available closer and faster to the patients. Factors of success were active involvement of the project participants, including primary care physicians at service locations, patient demand in services, technology that enabled delivery of services at acceptable quality, and good clinical methodology.

3.1 Clinical Methods

Functionally, telehomecare in ophthalmology is comprised of the following service levels:

- Patient evaluation and remote diagnostic services.
- Consultation leading to treatment.
- Continuous virtual medical supervision/monitoring.
- Clinical decision support, including automated diagnostics, computer technologies such as artificial intelligence.

The main ophthalmic diseases (from presbyopic correction till cataract, glaucoma, and AMD) correlate to patients age, and the main changes developing blindness manifests in elderly people. Furthermore, the hardest changes frequently develop in patients with hard general condition, unable to move to the ophthalmologist.

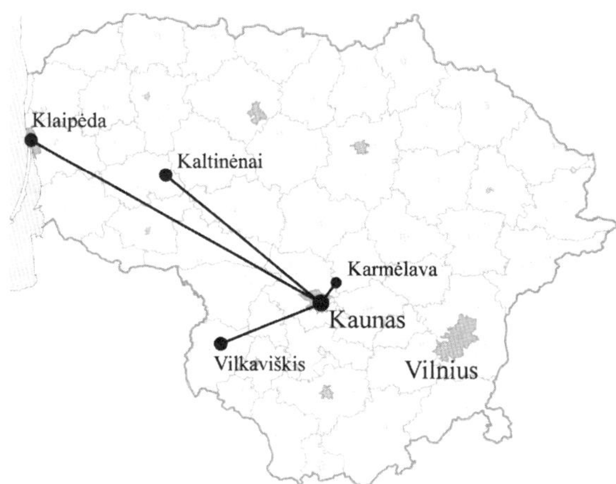

Fig. 1 Service locations

3.2 Project Participants

Stratelus, a small enterprise, a telenetwork coordinator, and service provider (competence center) has partnered with the Telemedicine Center, the Family Clinic, and the Department of Ophthalmology of Institute for Biomedical Research of the Lithuanian University of Health Sciences; Optomed OY, Oulu, Finland; and Remote Analysis OY, Helsinki, Finland in development of the telenetwork and service offering. The participants in remote areas whose patients were served were the Primary Health Care Center of Klasco (Klaipedos juru kroviniu kompanija—Klaipeda Stevedoring Company), Family Health Care Center of Vilkaviskis; Primary Health Care Center of Kaltinenai; Primary Health Care Center of JSC Elinta (Karmelava).

There were no specific requirements for the project participants—general requirements being interested and committed in participating in the project and telenetwork and willingness to learn using new technologies such as digital fundus camera and on-line data transmission.

3.3 Population Groups and Beneficiaries

The telenetwork was established in 4 remote areas with different distances from the Stratelus competence center which is based in Kaunas: Karmelava (20 km from Kaunas), Vilkaviskis (70 km), Kaltinenai (123 km), Klaipeda (205 km) (Fig. 1). Selection of the patients was done by family doctors and paramedics. Part of the selected patients was served at their home, part—in family clinic near their home (within local community).

Population groups have been selected in a number of rural areas in Lithuania. Among them, there were 2 groups—healthy people, who were subjected to screening, or preventive health check-up, and patients—people with clinical symptoms, who were subjected to monitoring. Focus was on 3 clinical conditions at this stage—diabetic retinopathy and age-related macula degeneration and glaucoma.

The project had not received any public funding. Some donations and in-kind contribution was received from several healthcare/pharmaceutical companies. The reasons of participants' interest in this project were ability to expand their services to their patients (their access to high competence diagnostics); by providing their patients with better and more timely diagnostics, decrease possibility of acute diseases or complications when treatment can be more complicated and more costly; develop their competence in ophthalmology. The ultimate beneficiary is the patient—it can be noted that accessibility of patients in remote locations to high competence diagnostics is constrained by such factors as distance to competence centre; wait time; travel time and resources; patient mobility; determination. Bringing service and experts to patients' home or to a distance minimal to their home (most of patients that were served in family clinics live within 10 min) from their home or work place.

3.4 Methodology and Implementation

The methodology of screening was based on the need for collecting the data and information needed for patient evaluation.

Screening was performed by tertiary level specialists. They made the choice on which tertiary level tests that are not available at primary level are necessary. This choice could not be made by a primary level physician. Thus, there was a selection of patients made at the screening—those who need to travel to a competence centre for more complex tests and evaluation and/or for surgery, and those who can be diagnosed locally. In addition, tertiary level specialists-ophthalmologists trained primary care/family physicians on working with the digital diagnostic handheld equipment suitable for telemedicine, acquisition and transmission of data to the competence centre for consultation and evaluation. With active involvement and relevant training of primary care physicians, remote diagnostics will enable diagnosis be made remotely for a large proportion of patient population.

3.5 Technological Innovative Elements

The most recent version of a Smartscope digital handheld eye fundus camera was used (Fig. 3), and a specialized software was used for online data transmission which was enabled by availability of fast data networks.

3.6 Patient Recruitment, Dissemination, and Screening Process

Patients for screening at remote locations were identified, selected, and recruited by participating primary care/family physicians or paramedics. The information dissemination about the project to the patients was based on direct contacts between the local medical staff and patients. Most of the primary care physicians, nurses have lived in the area for a long time and know their location and people very well. This also helped to maintain trust between patients and physicians in offering new service. Based on multiple factors including patient condition, some of the patients were assigned consultation at home, some—in the near proximity to home, or at their workplace.

Though physically screening was performed at primary level facility, methodology, and technology used included tertiary level such as ultrasound which was performed by tertiary level ophthalmologists. Our findings were that in homecare environment, a combination of trained primary care/family physicians or nurses and innovative telemedicine diagnostic technologies, such as handheld ophthalmoscopes, and transmitting the data for evaluation to competence centre, it is possible to provide sufficiently precise diagnosis without having a patient to travel to a tertiary level medical facility. Thus, homecare can effectively bring high quality healthcare closer to a patient and decrease the time to diagnosis.

There were 2 groups of patients:

- Patients who arrived for evaluation to a clinic near their home (within 10 min travel) or at their workplace.
- Patients located beyond 10 min from a clinic, or patients with impaired mobility were evaluated at home.

Evaluation at a primary care clinic was performed by physicians-ophthalmologists who arrived from a competence centre. Their aim was to perform the first screenings and train local medical personnel, including the use of handheld equipment for ophthalmology. The investigation included basic ophthalmological examination, measurement of intraocular pressure, biomicroscopy by a slit lamp and eye fundus photography by handheld digital fundus camera. Some of the tests were performed by a family doctor or nurse with participation and observation of an ophthalmologist from the competence centre.

Evaluation at the patient's home was performed by a family doctor or nurse with participation and observation of an ophthalmologist from the competence centre using the handheld camera Smartscope with add-ons for fundus photography and anterior eye segment investigation. Investigation included measurement of visual acuity, tonometry, slit lamp examination, Schirmer's test, dilation of the pupil, and eye fundus examination with Volk 90D lens, eye fundus photography (digital handheld eye fundus camera Smartscope, Figs. 2 (right picture) and 3) and data transmitting. Cup disk ratio of the optic nerve head was also evaluated. The data obtained—visual materials i.e., pictures and patient data—were transmitted to the Stratelus competence centre for processing and evaluation by highly skilled

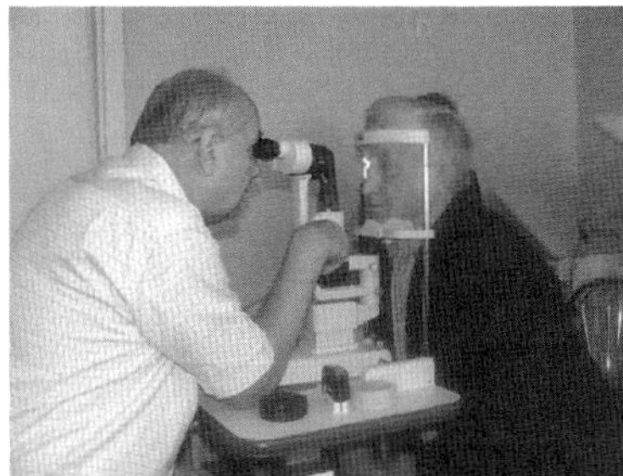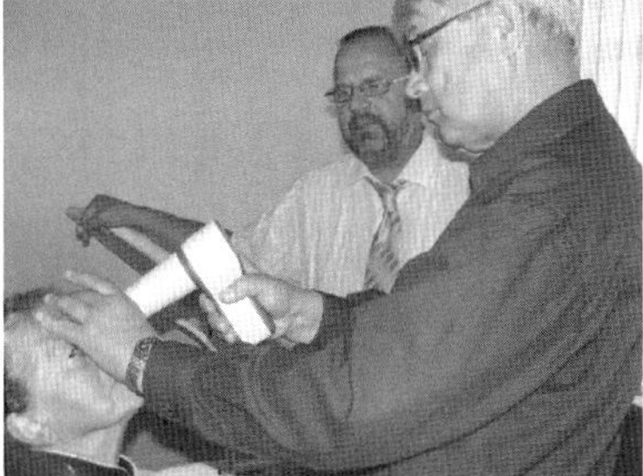

Fig. 2 Patient screening at the Kaltinenai primary care center. Digital eye fundus camera use is shown on the *right* picture

Fig. 3 Handheld digital eye fundus camera (Courtesy of Optomed OY)

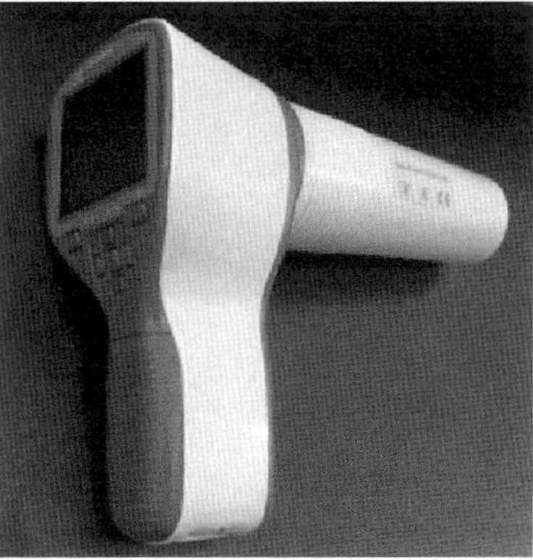

ophthalmologist. The focus of diagnostics in home and primary care environment was preliminary diagnosis and identification of the need for further action. Technical aspects are covered in the chapter below.

3.7 Patient—Competence Centre Interface: Data Transmission, Remote Analysis

The equipment used was a digital handheld eye fundus camera together with specialized software for telenetworking and image exchange. Patient fundus images acquired while visiting them at home or at a participating family clinic were sent by local family physicians/general practitioners to the competence center of Stratelus where they were evaluated by tertiary level specialist physicians and evaluation results with clinical recommendations were sent back to the local family physicians. The data processing, transmitting and evaluation process and tools are shown in Figs. 3, 4, 5, 6 and 7.

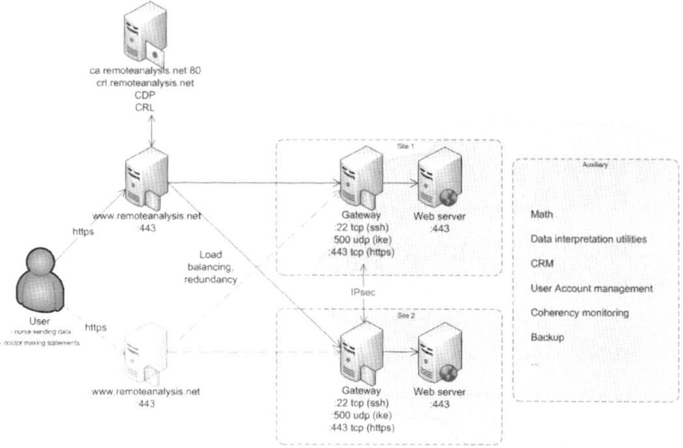

Fig. 4 Data processing (Courtesy of Remote Analysis)

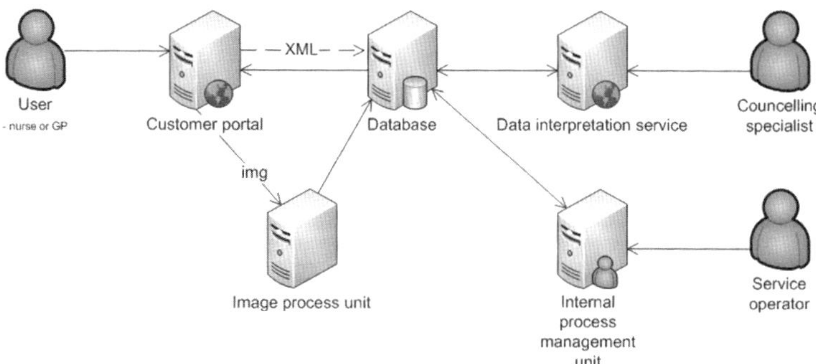

Fig. 5 Data transmitting

3.8 Clinical Findings

The main result of the screenings was provision of timely and high competence diagnostics that was enabled by competence of the physicians (experienced ophthalmologists from the Lithuanian University of Health Sciences), high quality portable equipment, and local cooperation.

The screenings provided with valuable clinical and organizational experience. We noticed direct relationship between remoteness (distance from competence centre) and health condition (occurrence and complexity of diseases) which we believe to a large extent is caused by time, resource and mobility constraints.

Another relationship was age-based: elderly population which is more prevalent in remote rural areas is more likely to show age related diseases, their complications, such as blood vessels blockage, retinal detachment, age-related macula

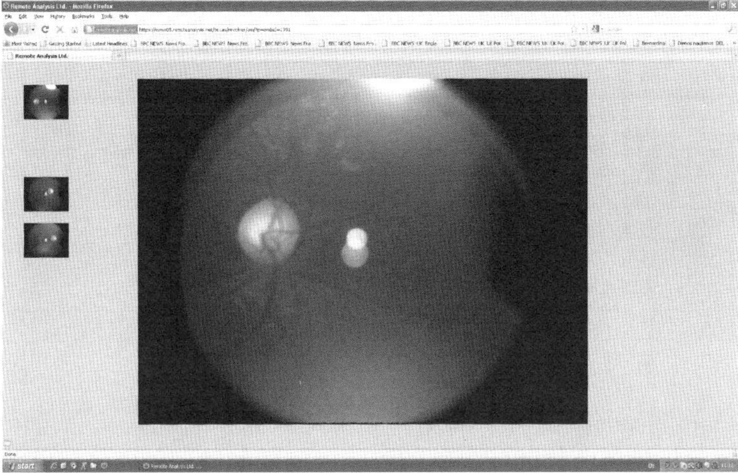

Fig. 6 Screen (display) of transmission from patients' end to competence center via remote analysis software. The second picture of four pictures sent is enlarged

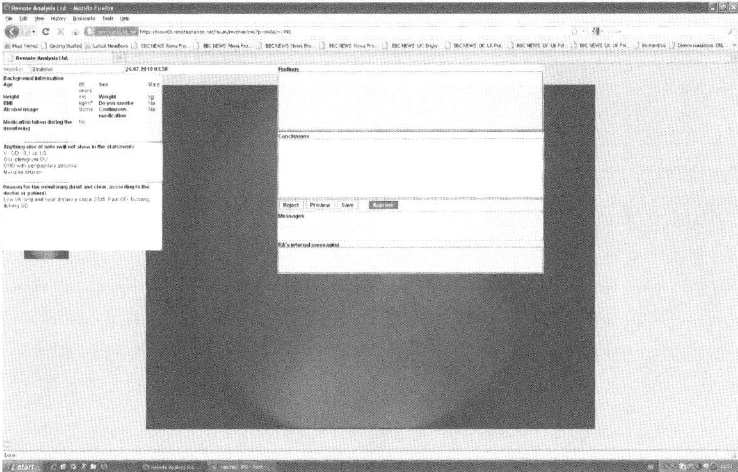

Fig. 7 Screen (display) at the competence center prepared for expert decision to send. Patient data field is visible on the *left side*; field for expert's response/evaluation is visible in the middle of the screen

degeneration. This, in turn, further decreases patients' mobility which makes accessibility to health care even more constrained. High patient turnout at the locations involved demonstrated that homecare or near-homecare is in high demand and can significantly increase patients' accessibility to health services. Patients' distribution by age and gender are shown in Table 1. There was no

Table 1 Patients' distribution by location, age, and gender

Age group	Location				Total
	Klaipėda	Karmėlava	Vilkaviškis	Kaltinėnai	
15–20	2/1 (3)	0/0 (0)	0/0 (0)	2/1 (3)	4/2 (6)
21–30	2/2 (4)	6/5 (11)	2/0 (2)	2/0 (2)	12/7 (19)
31–40	3/5 (8)	9/15 (24)	1/1 (2)	2/0 (2)	15/21 (36)
41–50	6/4 (10)	16/11 (27)	2/1 (3)	4/5 (9)	28/21 (49)
51–60	5/4 (9)	8/3	3/2	6/6	22/15 (37)
61–70	1/0 (1)	1/1	2/2	4/8	8/11 (19)
>70	0/1 (1)	1/0	0/2	3/4	4/7 (11)
Total	19/17 (36)	41/35 (76)	10/8 (18)	23/24 (47)	93/84 (177)

significant differentiation by gender and the patient population generally corresponded with the general population trends.

Table 2 shows patient distribution by disease. We could not compare frequency of diseases with the statistical average frequency of diseases of Lithuania because patients were chosen selectively and reflect the spectrum of diseases that telehomecare could potentially address. Furthermore, some patients had 2 or 3 diseases such as Cataract, Glaucoma, and dacryocystitis. This was in line with our aim to pilot and utilize telehomecare opportunities. There was a significant number of patients with refractive errors (Myopia, Hyperopia, Astigmatism) which we did not address within the scope of telehomecare.

3.9 Clinical Conditions Investigated

Glaucoma is one of the main ophthalmological problems in the elderly population in Lithuania. There are about 10–12% of all patients suffering from glaucoma and many people with suspected glaucoma. Most important diagnostic sign of glaucoma is evaluation of optic nerve head cupping and it's dynamics. Traditionally, it is a complicated test, which needs to be performed correctly in an ophthalmologists office, at least equipped with slit lamp and 90D fundus lens, and dilated pupil, what sometimes is contraindicated for glaucoma patients. For the evaluation of the optic nerve head cupping as a homecare procedure, we used non-mydriatic (narrow pupil) digital eye fundus camera, operated by nurse together with rutin tonometry at patients home, and transmitted the image to teleophthalmology competence center for processing and evaluation.

Diabetic retinopathy was the second focal clinical condition. On average, out of 10 patients with diabetic retinopathy, 2 were seen at home, eye fundus images of 2 patients were sent to the competence centre for consultation regarding laser treatment. Diabetic retinopathy is another disease that poses considerable challenges to ophthalmologists and general practitioners. It is the second most prevalent cause of blindness in Lithuania. Its diagnostics and treatment is

Table 2 Clinical findings of screening

Diagnosis	Location				Total
	Klaipėda	Karmėlava	Vilkaviškis	Kaltinėnai	
Cataract (beginning)	11	18	8	27	64
Cataract (surgical)	1	2	3	6	12
Glaucoma compensated	5	2	2	4	13
Glaucoma subcompensated	0	0	2	3	5
Glaucoma suspected	3	2	2	3	10
Glaucoma secondary traumatic				1	1
Dry eye	0	12	4	8	24
AMD (dry)	6	8	6	12	32
AMD (wet)	0	0	1	3	4
Diabetic retinopathy	1	3	2	4	10
Corneal opacities (leucoma)	0	0	1	2	2
Anterior uveitis	0	0	1	2	3
Keratitis e lagophthalmo	0	0	1	0	1
Conjunctivitis	0	1	0	1	2
Chalazion	0	0	1	0	1
Refraction error	15	23	6	12	56
High complicated myopia	0	2	0	1	3
Optic nerve disease	1				1
Retinal peripheral degeneration	0	1	2	1	4
Preretinal fibrosis			1	1	2
Dacryocystitis	0	0	0	1	1
Healthy	0	11	0	1	12

concentrated at the 5 largest cities of Lithuania and patients are supposed to go there. However, the number of patients coming for regular evaluation to one of those 5 centers is significantly decreasing with the increase of distance to the center. It is related to the mobility of patients and accessibility to local public transportation. Homecare is a solution that could potentially avert this trend and improve clinical outcomes.

Age related macular degeneration—third target in our screening. It's frequency correlates with age. However, it was observed to appear at a younger age as well. There were 36 such patients at the screening. For most of them, dry form was diagnosed, which requires follow-up—but the good news is that it can be performed remotely. Only 2 wet forms were diagnosed—those patients had to be referred to the tertiary centre for treatment.

3.10 Images Processing and Assessment

The assessment of digital pictures of eye fundus is one the most relevant and frequently used methods for diagnosis of glaucoma, diabetic retinopathy, and age related macular degeneration. It is more easily mastered, accessible, and

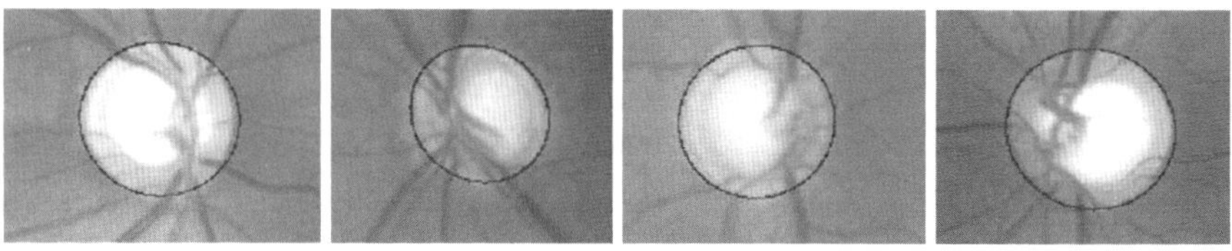

Fig. 8 Images of optical nerve heads with elliptical approximation (gold standard)

inexpensive compared with laser methods (HRT and OCT). For diagnosis and evaluation of glaucoma changes the ONH digital pictures still stay as golden standard [15–17].

Screenings usually result in a high quantity of eye fundus images and their evaluation sometimes becomes complex purely because of the volume, when healthy images have to be distinguished from unhealthy—which have to be evaluated by an experienced expert-physician.

In order to increase efficiency and enable processing of high volume of clinical information, together with the Vilnius Mathematics and Informatics Institute, we started development of automatic eye fundus parametrisation methods. The first one we chose for parametrisation was optic nerve head and its cupping [18–21].

The main advantage of the proposed automatic optical nerve disk localization and approximation method is that the location of the optical nerve head is found automatically without involvement of the physician. Below is a brief scheme of the elliptical automatic optical nerve head localization and approximation. The method consists of the following steps:

- Step 1. Initial image processing.
- Step 2. Localisation of the optical nerve head. Identification of margins.
- Step 3. Elliptical automatic optical nerve head approximation.
- Step 4. Optic nerve head cupping approximation.

Samples of elliptical automatic optical nerve head approximation are shown in Fig. 8, cupping approximation—Fig. 9.

Although the image quality of the handheld camera is lower than taken with professional stationary camera (gold standard), it was sufficient to recognize optic nerve cupping in glaucoma (Fig. 8), hard exudates and hemmorages in nonproliferative diabetic retinopathy. A shortcoming of the version of the camera used was in recognition of early stages of age related degeneration when only small macular edema can persist. The comparison of the output by the handheld camera and gold standard (stationary camera) resulted in giving the handheld camera a score of 7 as compared to score of 10 for the gold standard (Fig. 10). As in the methodology that was used, this camera was used especially to help general practitioners in screening and selecting patients for ophthalmologist's consultation, the quality of image was found to be sufficient for this purpose. The overall clinical advantages in providing patients with better and faster access to services were significant.

Fig. 9 Optic nerve head and cupping automatic approximation and parameterization (image made with digital handheld eye fundus camera)

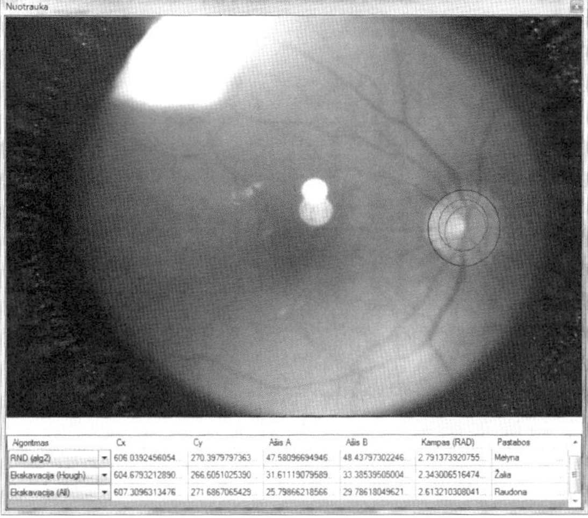

Fig. 10 Eye fundus image taken with the handheld fundus camera

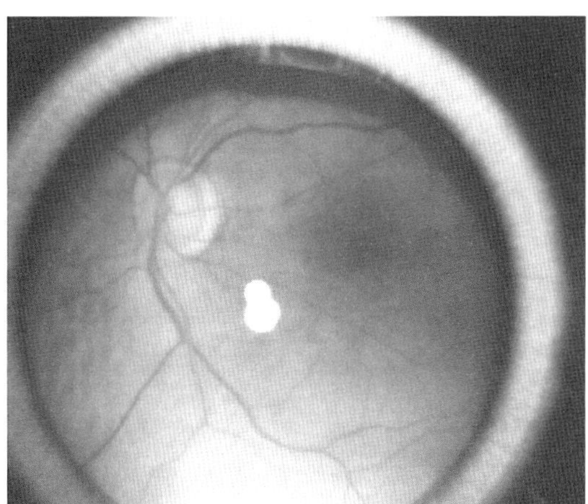

4 Internal Influences on Development and Outcome

As we noted, factors of project success were active involvement of the project participants, including primary care physicians at service locations, patient demand in services, technology that enabled delivery of services at acceptable quality, and good clinical methodology. Active participants of the project were local/primary care physicians, tertiary level physicians, project leader and coordinator, and patients. Motivation of all the participants was maintained by expected outcome of the project, successful offering of health care services delivery in a home environment. In terms of the number of project participants, the project was small (in the range of 15–20 physicians and in the range of 200 patients) which made project management and coordination and interaction between the physicians simple and effective. Project participants were required to

Table 3 Comparison of costs between telehomecare and visit to tertiary healthcare facility

Average service cost at remote location, LTL/EUR	Remote location	Distance to competence centre, km	Average patient travel time, h	Average patient travel cost, LTL/EUR single	Average patient transportation cost, return ticket, and accompanying person LTL/EUR	Average service cost at competence centre, LTL/EUR[a]
70/20	Kaltinenai	123	3	29.5/9	118/34	72/20
70/20	Vilkaviskis	70	2	24/7	96/28	72/20
70/20	Karmelava, Elinta	20	1	3.5/1	14/4	72/20
70/20	Klaipeda	205	4	53/15	212/61	72/20

[a] Average wait for in-person consultation at the Eye Clinic of the Lithuanian University of Health Sciences is 1 month

keep their commitment—local/primary care physicians, learn the technology, interact with their patients, explain, make appointments, participate in clinical decision making; tertiary level physicians—to keep commitment provide with clinical support, evaluate images, consult. We found high enthusiasm of especially rural physicians who were motivated also by learning and using new technologies which are often limited to urban clinics or hospitals are not always reach the periphery. The tertiary level physicians found it motivating to diagnose patients earlier than they would be if they had to come for a live visit to a tertiary level hospital, however their time availability needs to be well considered when planning as they often have busy agendas in academic and clinical activities.

5 External Influences on Development and Outcome

5.1 Economic Aspects

We found that there was an economic benefit of providing care at home or next to home. We saw that physician's time can be used very efficiently when performing screening and seeing high number of patients per hour. Efficient distribution of roles and tasks and inclusion of local primary care physicians and nursing staff for some parts of the process adds up to the efficiency.

Significant advantage to a patient comes from travel time and cost savings. As can be seen from Table 3, average service cost when providing serviced at home or near home is 20 EUR/patient, while an option of traveling to the tertiary centre, depending on distance, may reach up to 81 EUR. Even in case of the closest location, there is some cost advantage (4 EUR/patient) and definitely time advantage. When estimating average travel time and cost, we assumed public transportation is used and we took into consideration wait times for public transportation.

Table 4 Kaiser Permanente study (1997) [22, 23]

Variable	In person	Telehealth[a]
Number of visits/day	5.2	15–20
Time of visit (min)	45	18
Travel	Yes	No
Reimbursement for travel	Yes	No
Time from triage to when patient is seen	24–48 h	Few minutes

Savings of 33–50% were noted

[a] Researchers noted that with telehealth the patient could be seen many times in 1 day if needed

Economic benefit for a participating local primary care clinic comes in the form of extended services to their patients and, by potentially decreasing occurrence of late or complicated diagnosis (although we haven't had sufficient statistical data to prove it), costs of care may be saved as well. In our screenings, we saw trends generally similar to the ones shown in other sources [22–24] (Table 4).

5.2 The Impact of Project Outcome on Project Partners

The positive impact of the project and its viability provided all project participants with motivation to continue the project. Although there was a role of economic benefits in this, interest to continue was driven by clinical and learning reasons— the project helped to meet patient demand in services at rural and remote locations and it provided the participating physicians with opportunities to learn, clinically and use of new method and technologies.

6 User Aspects

(a) *Synergies and efficiency*: Several synergies evolved in the course of the project: local/primary care physicians—tertiary level physicians; local physicians— patients; local physicians—residents practicing in family clinics—the university residents belong to. All these synergies have positive impact on the idea, structure, and outcome of the project. Likewise, motivation and involvement of all these parties is important to keep such a project going. From an organizational point of view, the project demonstrated improvement of efficiency as there was considerable preparation for the screening visits at remote locations, good sharing of functions between the medical staff participating in patient visits, which resulted into a higher number of patients seen per hour than in a normal office visit setting. Synergies that developed via close cooperation between the team of the tertiary level physicians and local primary care physicians also contributed to increased efficiency and clinical quality. By participating in the project and in patient encounters, competence of local primary care physicians has been steadily increasing which helped to strengthen cooperation and professional ties between project participants and achieve a high level of understanding and integration. This will be used for further improvements and project expansion.

(b) *Education*: Training of the primary care physicians on innovative diagnostic medical technologies and equipment and using it in remote locations can decrease the number of unnecessary referrals to the tertiary level facilities, and to make diagnostics sooner and avoid complications. Training and involvement of the primary level physicians in telehealthcare also increases their professional competence which is an important benefit to the healthcare system. Another component is use of telehomecare in training the residents practicing in family clinics, that is an additional educational tool helping to develop their clinical competence, and also a tool to train use new technologies. In the long term, they will more likely adopt telemedicine in their practice.

(c) *Challenges*: Both the ultimate users—the patients, and primary care clinics as intermediary service users demonstrated high level of satisfaction in the outcomes of the project. There were several challenges that we experienced:

- Appropriate training had to be provided to the participating primary care physicians and nursing staff, such as use of Smartscope for acquiring eye fundus images, online data transmission. Specifically, obtaining the highest quality eye fundus images takes not only high quality equipment, but also training and experience of an investigator, and training is still ongoing for most of the participating primary care physicians. The training is provided by the tertiary level ophthalmologists.
- Seeing patients at home was some organizational and psychological, to a patient, challenge—tertiary level physicians are generally not visiting patients at home often so it required a little different organizational approach, and also, in a screening setting, going to see patients from home to home involves some extra time spent for travel. On the other hand, not all patients felt comfortable by receiving a team of physicians at home for screenings rather than emergency visits, although they were happy with the service they received.

User satisfaction and user-friendliness were important factor in project success. The service was accepted by patients and physicians and demonstrated high satisfaction. Looking to the future, however, training and experience of participating primary care physicians will be an essential factor in ensuring the data transmitted to the tertiary level has good quality, therefore they need to receive appropriate training on using the technologies that are used in the project.

(d) *Legal Aspects*: There were no legal aspects in the course of this project as in all occasions there was a live presence of a physician at a patient encounter. However, moving forward, when technology and training allows trained nurses or paramedics to acquire and transmit eye images to the tertiary level for evaluation, legal aspects of responsibility and liability insurance as well as service reimbursement will become critical and may become an impediment, if not addressed.

7 General Aspects

Implementation of the project and its continuation will contribute to the quality of life of communities in rural and remote areas. Mobility of patients in those locations are often limited by physical and sometimes behavioral, psychological reasons and providing them with better access to healthcare is a step ahead not only making those areas more livable to elderly population but also more attractive for younger generation. As telehomecare is not a mandated service and has not yet become a prevailing or even significant mode of health care services delivery yet, initiative and willingness cooperate is crucial for the model to work. Resolution of legal (including the aspects of physicians' liability), quality of services, and financial aspects is important if we want this model to be sustainable. Local communities will be interested in receiving better services closer to patients, but it is important to assure quality and maintain trust in this model. Patient/community outreach was mainly based on direct contacts by local physicians who usually know their community very well, and to some extent, local press.

8 Conclusion

The aim of our project was to test and pilot the ways and methods of improving accessibility of population in rural and remote locations to high quality and timely healthcare in a real clinical setting. Population in those locations (in terms of accessibility of their population to high quality health care services) is often underserved by modern diagnostic services, largely due to the travel time, cost and wait time constraints. Bringing the service closer to the patients, their home or near home serves as an equivalent of virtually providing tertiary level service at a primary level physical location. This project has improved accessibility to advanced diagnostics and timely healthcare for a number of rural population who otherwise would often choose not, or could not to, travel to tertiary level health-care providers for advanced diagnostics until late stage of symptoms. By using telehomecare, we did not completely replace the need for some patients to visit the tertiary clinic in person—it complemented each other, allowed to eliminate some unnecessary visits to the tertiary level clinic, and in some cases, encouraged patients to visit the tertiary level clinic and address their health condition sooner.

The available technology represents the strength of this type of service, and in the light of general technology trends, further improvements in deliverables (e.g., image quality) and cost should be expected in near term. The opportunity is represented by demand in access to health care services at acceptable costs which would improve the quality of life in rural or remote communities not only for the prevailing elderly population but to younger generation as well. The challenges and threats that we identified were—conservative approach to new modes in physician–patient interaction such as telemedicine from physicians and from patients, and legal and financial (payment for service) basis for telemedicine that is lagging behind. Telemedicine is still a new method for the wider public and it also has a psychological aspect of direct physician–patient interaction. Our project has shown many of those telehomecare benefits to a patient, health professional, and healthcare payer that were already shown by other studies and sources, such as, improved access to health professional, patients can be seen quicker, be seen more often, stay home longer before becoming institutionalized, patients can be kept in the community (which can show savings), but specifically, we have shown that in ophthalmology, big potential in homecare and telemedicine is being opened by introduction of high quality imaging devices such as handheld fundus/anterior segment cameras because quality if image is the essential factor in making ophthalmological diagnosis.

The overall result of the project was success and it showed that initiation and delivery of small/medium telehomecare projects is possible, it can produce good clinical results, and they can be well received by all involved (patients, local physicians, tertiary level physicians), run on small budgets and have good chance to be self-sustainable in long-term. This will make this project into a continuous activity which we expect to expand significantly. There was a patient cost savings benefit demonstrated which would also translate into cost savings to the healthcare system in general, especially when telemedicine/telehomecare expands to more communities, runs on continuous basis, and addresses preventive screenings and chronic disease treatment to large part of a population. Factors contributing to project success were active involvement of the project participants, including primary care physicians at service locations, patient demand in services, technology that enabled delivery of services at acceptable quality, and good clinical methodology.

The lessons learned were: necessity of having a high quality, portable, relatively low-cost equipment suitable for telemedicine applications; necessity of generating interest of such projects among local family physicians; necessity of proper training of local family physicians in using the equipment and telemedicine applications; self-sustainability is not easy in the times of economic–financial stress but on a broad-scale, it is beneficial both for the family physicians and patients.

References

1. Paunksnis A, Barzdžiukas V, Lukoševičius M, Kurapkienė S, Almquist L-O, Severgardh P. Teleophthalmology for second opinion and clinical decision support. Proceedings in the 2nd international conference "ehealth in Common Europe". Krakow (Poland) 11–12 March, 2003:61.
2. Iakovidis I, Purcarea O. eHealth in Europe: from vision to reality. eHealth: combining Health telematics, telemedicine, biomedical engineering, and bioinformatics to the edge. Amsterdam: IOS Press; 2008. p. 163–168.
3. Balas AE, Krishna S, Tessema AT. eHealth: connecting health care and public health. eHealth: combining health telematics, telemedicine, biomedical engineering, and bioinformatics to the edge. Amsterdam: IOS Press; 2008. p. 169–176.
4. Ingram D. The journey of health informatics. Proceedings of International conference on e-health in common Europe. Krakow (Poland) June 5–6, 2003;3–18.

5. Duplaga M. Chronic care in e-world—the growing evidence. Proceedings of International conference on e-health in common Europe. Krakow (Poland) June 5–6, 2003;43–61.
6. Winnem OM, Walderhaug S. Distributed, role-based, guideline-based desicion support. Proceedings of International conference on e-health in common Europe. Krakow (Poland) June 5–6, 2003;101–109.
7. Adeyinka M. The trans-European telemedicine initiative (TETI). Proceedings of International conference on e-health in common Europe. Krakow (Poland) June 5–6, 2003:261–269.
8. Paunksnis A, Barzdžiukas V, Kurapkienė S. Teleophthalmology in Lithuania. In: Yogesan K, Kumar S, Goldschmidt L, Cuadros J, editors. Teleophthalmology. Berlin: Springer; 2006; chapter 22:167–177.
9. European Comision Cordis. Health research available in http://cordis.europa.eu/fp7/health/home_en.html.
10. Thede LQ, Sewell J. Carrying healthcare to the client. In Informatics and nursing: competences and application. 2009 Chapter 22. Available in http://www.telehealth.ca/intrototelehomecare.html.
11. Chanwimaluang T, Fan G, Fransen SR. Correction to "Hybrid retinal image registration". IEEE transactions on information technology in biomedicine. 2007; November 11:110–110.
12. Choong YF, Rakebrandt F, North RV, Morgan JE. Acutance, an objective measure of retinal nerve fibre image clarity. Br J Ophthalmol. 2003;87:322–6.
13. Fleming AD, Philip S, Goatman KA, Olson JA, Sharp PF. Automated assessment of diabetic retinal image quality based on clarity and field definition. Invest Ophthalmol Vis Sci. 2006;47(3):1120–5.
14. Jonas JB, Mardin ChY, Grundler AE. Comparison of measurements of neuroretinal rim area between confocal laser scanning tomography and planimetry of photographs. Brit J Ophthalmol. 1998;82:362–6.
15. Lalonde M, Gagnon L, Boucher M. Automatic visual quality assessment in optical fundus images. Proceedings of Vision Interface. Ottawa, Ontario, Canada; 2001:259–264.
16. Neubauer AS, Krieglstein TR, Chryssafis C, Thiel M, Kampik A. Comparison of optical coherence tomography and fundus photography for measuring the optic disc size. 2006; 26:13–8.
17. Niemeijer M, van Ginneken B, Russell SR, Suttorp-Schulten MSA, Abràmoff MD. Automated detection and differentiation of drusen, exudates, and cotton-wool spots in digital color fundus photographs for diabetic retinopathy diagnosis. Invest Ophthalmol Vis Sci. 2007;48(5):2260–7.
18. Treigys P, Dzemyda G, Barzdžiukas V. Automated positioning of overlapping eye fundus images. ICCS. 2008;1:770–9.
19. Treigys P, Šaltenis V, Dzemyda G, Barzdžiukas V, Paunksnis A. Automated optic nerve disc parameterization. Informatica. 2008;19(3):403–20.
20. Bernatavičienė J, Dzemyda G, Kurasova O, Buteikienė D, Barzdžiukas V, Paunksnis A. Rule induction for ophthalmological data classification, Proceedings of EURO Mini Conference on Continuous Optimization and Knowledge-Based Technologies, Vilnius, Technika; 2008; 328–334.
21. Treigys P, Šaltenis V. Neural network as an ophthalmologic disease classifier. Inf Tech Cont. 2007;36(4):365–71.
22. Johnston B, Wheeler L, Deuser J. Tele-Home Health: Kaiser Permanente Medical Center's Pilot Project. Telemedicine Today, July 1997.
23. Johnston B, Wheeler L, Deuser J, Sousa KH. Outcomes of the Kaiser Permanente Tele-Home Health Research Project. Arch Fam Med 2000;9(1):40–45.
24. Elford R. An introduction to telehome care. Available at http://www.telehealth.ca/intrototelehomecare.html.

Implementation of Mobile Computing in Canadian Homecare Programs: Project Risk Management and its Influence on Project Success

Claude Sicotte and Guy Paré

Abstract Mobile computing is one of a growing number of information technologies applied in the context of homecare services. While home telemonitoring enables clinical interventions *at a distance*, mobile computing allows clinicians to integrate the care process *on site* at the patient's home. As digital homecare is a fairly recent phenomenon and our understanding of the challenges and barriers associated with its implementation is still in its infancy, we used a clinical information system risk analysis framework to investigate how project risk management of mobile computing implementations was applied and how it shaped a project's outcome. We followed the ongoing development and implementation of a mobile computing project in real time at nine homecare program sites in the Province of Québec, Canada. We analyzed each site's implementation strategy, i.e., the pre-existing and emergent risks, the risk mitigation strategies aimed at eliminating the hindering factors and at favoring successful outcomes at each site. In studying the relations between the various elements (implementation strategy, risk occurrence, and level of success), we were able to draw a series of lessons to help decrease failures and further the success of mobile computing in homecare programs.

Keywords Mobile computing · Homecare · Implementation · Project risk management

C. Sicotte (✉)
Department of Health Administration, University of Montreal, P.O. Box 6128,
Downtown Station, Montreal, QC H3C 3J7, Canada
e-mail: Claude.Sicotte@umontreal.ca

G. Paré
HEC Montréal, Montreal, Canada
e-mail: Guy.Pare@hec.ca

Commun Med Care Compunetics (2011) 3: 89–113
DOI: 10.1007/8754_2011_24
© Springer-Verlag Berlin Heidelberg 2011
Published Online: 11 May 2011

1 Introduction

Population ageing is a global phenomenon affecting most regions of the world. Among OECD member countries, over 40% of total health spending is already being used to manage patients 65 years of age and older [19]. As we age, the incidence and prevalence of chronic diseases increase. This increased burden of chronic disease on health care resources and the resulting costs are a powerful incentive for finding effective ways to care for these patients. Further, in light of the increasing shortage of health care providers, especially outside large urban areas, the challenge has become even more complex in many developed countries. In response, many governments acknowledge the importance of providing homecare services. In fact, expanding the range of health care services provided in the home—one of the recommendations recently made by the World Health Organization [32]—is part of a fundamental trend observed in many health systems, including those in Canada, the United States, and many European countries [33].

Information technology applied to clinical information systems (CIS) is perceived as a key enabler for the implementation of these changes [17, 34]. New delivery mechanisms, such as telehomecare—defined as the application of information and communication technologies to bring health care to the home environment—are emphasizing care in the patient's home as an alternative to acute care and as a complement to primary care. We identified two generic forms of digital homecare. Under the first model, called home telemonitoring, patients utilize condition-specific devices to monitor their clinical condition [23, 24]. Various technological devices such as personal digital assistants (PDAs), cellular phones, or PCs are then used to transmit information to a central telehealth management system which collects, stores, and displays clinical data and assessment documentation. Clinicians then utilize provider-focused devices to access the data associated with a cohort of patients and to provide timely interventions.

A second form of digital homecare model, called mobile computing, targets providers, not patients, as its main users and allows, on site or elsewhere, clinical data management visit scheduling, care planning and data sharing [4, 22]. The variety of mobile devices used by clinicians includes personal digital assistants (PDAs), laptops, tablet computers, GPS, and smartphones, to name but a few [11, 28]. These devices can access clinical information from a distance or update in real time the patient record or care plan. This also facilitates continuity and coordination of care among the care team. While home telemonitoring enables clinical interventions *at a distance*, this second form of mobile computing allows clinicians to integrate the care process *on site* at the patient's home.

The present study concerns the second form of digital homecare. It examines the deployment and success of a large mobile computing project which took place in nine homecare units located in Québec, Canada. As digital homecare is a fairly new phenomenon and our understanding of the challenges and barriers associated with digital homecare implementation projects is still in its infancy, we used a CIS risk analysis framework [25] to investigate how project risk management was applied and how it shaped project outcomes.

2 Background

Overall, research performed on various forms of remote medicine (called tele-medicine or telehealth) has yielded mixed results as much with respect to its acceptance by targeted users as to its difficulty in harnessing intended benefits [17, 18]. Indeed, several systematic reviews have reported mixed findings with respect to clinical outcomes, clinical processes, healthcare utilization, and costs e.g., [8, 14].

The vast majority of studies targeting digital homecare have mostly looked at the first generic model, that is to say home telemonitoring. Some systematic reviews which analyzed the effects associated with home telemonitoring have been published. In short, these reviews have shown that home telemonitoring of chronic diseases represents an effective patient management approach that can produce accurate and reliable data, empower patients, influence their attitude and behavior, and potentially improve their medical condition [6, 7, 20, 23, 24]. However, benefits vary greatly according to pathologies, and research methods used to study these effects are often weak.

Contrary to the extant literature on home telemonitoring, there is a paucity of research on mobile computing. The few scientific studies we found addressed two main themes. On the one hand, two studies analyzed what determines mobile healthcare systems acceptance by healthcare professionals. The first of these studies indicated that system compatibility, perceived usefulness and perceived ease of use significantly affected healthcare professional behavioral intent [35]. The second collected the opinions of nurses who had used personal digital assistants for 1 month in their daily activities. Data analysis revealed that nurses' perception of usefulness is the main factor in the adoption of mobile technology [37]. On the other hand, three studies were aimed at analyzing the benefits to be gained by mobile computing applications. The first study, which focused on return-on-investment analysis prior to system development, indicated a potential net savings on tangible costs [1]. Another study pertaining to a point-of-care home hospice information system showed that the new system allowed marginal efficiency gains, but it enabled improvements in the quality of point-of-care services [13]. The last study showed improvements in productivity with respect to the number of patients treated for CODP as well as the number of visits performed per shift and encompassing the number of direct hours of care provided in patients' homes [22].

Despite its apparent attractiveness, homecare mobile computing is faced with two typical challenges: gaining targeted user acceptance and achieving intended benefits. These two challenges must be resolved if mobile computing is to survive and is to be dispensed in the health sector. The achievement of these outcomes implies important changes in provider and patient attitudes and behaviors, as well as a re-organization of professional work so as to adapt to this new form of care delivery. Due to its intrinsic characteristics, mobile computing, as well as the other forms of telehealth, results inevitably in the reconfiguration of existing work practices and in the emergence of new organizational forms. This new way of working is most likely to trigger a variety of shifts in administrative mechanisms, work processes, and power relationships. The present study strives to better understand how these technological and organizational changes can be implemented successfully [2, 9, 16]. Such an endeavor requires a comprehensive framework for capturing a large spectrum of project risk factors that are likely to play a role in mobile computing success. The framework we used is described in the following section.

3 CIS Project Risk Taxonomy

Various impediments can slow down and even completely halt the implementation of CIS (including mobile technologies) in healthcare organizations. It is, therefore, imperative to adopt an analytical model to make sense of what can remain lists of a-theoretical factors. For this purpose, we used an analytical approach that is common to the information systems field: risk analysis [25]. This type of analysis transfers implementation impediments into a notion of risk which indicates a propensity/probability of negative results with respect to the project objectives and users' expectations. In order to identify the risk factors, we opted for a framework that is limited enough to distinguish the risk factors and broad enough to be comprehensive. We chose a risk taxonomy developed for the health sector following a Delphi study. This taxonomy identifies the risk factors that are common to implementation projects in CISs [21]. The model offers 30 risk factors which are classified into seven dimensions. The complete list of factors and dimensions included in the taxonomy is presented in Appendix 1.

The first dimension, technological risk (projects that fail to deliver operational systems) refers to hardware and software complexity. The key technology challenges in mobile technology continue to be the same as those which have characterized other technological advances over the past decades, namely, miniaturization, greater speed, and cost reduction [31]. Second, user risk (projects that fail to gain user acceptance) mainly refers to issues such as system adoption and resistance to change [15]. Third, usability risk (projects that fail to deliver proper functionalities) is related to the user-friendliness of the technological devices being deployed and the extent to which their functionalities are aligned with local tasks and practices. Task-technology fit has long been considered a critical success factor in both the information systems and medical informatics fields (e.g., [10, 29, 36]. Next, the project team risk dimension (projects that fail to bring together competent managers and project team members) refers to the lack of required skills, the ambiguity surrounding role definitions, and lack of strong project leadership. Fifth, project risk (projects that cannot meet their own budget, schedule or scope constraints) remains a common barrier in virtually all CIS projects [12]. Sixth, organization risk (projects that fail to gain enough organizational support) represents a significant barrier, especially when the organization is confronted with simultaneous organizational changes. Finally, the strategic/political risk dimension (projects that fail to build a strong enough political alliance) may be a difficult barrier to overcome in a context of extensive organizational change. In sum, such a project risk framework goes beyond the deterministic, magic bullet view in which technology is the sole factor of change. Rather, it reflects a sociotechnical approach that stresses the importance of a broader, multi-dimensional perspective [5].

In the present study, risk factors are defined as *contextual issues* that can influence the probability that an undesirable result will occur. Examples of undesirable results include missing deadlines, poor user adoption, and failing to achieve expected benefits. Risk factors are also considered as aspects upon which managers can act or intervene to various degrees by applying a series of palliative tactics (e.g., having future users help identify information requirements, managing relationships with external partners). According to such a contingent managerial view [2, 9], it is then possible to study project risks and their risk-mitigating managerial counteractions to understand their influence on project outcomes.

4 Methodology

4.1 Research Design and Settings

We carried out a multiple-case study of mobile computing in nine homecare units. These nine sites made use of the same technological solution between 2008 and 2010 and pursued similar goals. The two major objectives were the improvement of healthcare quality and that of nursing personnel productivity. The productivity improvement objective was particularly important to the Department of Health and the regional agencies which were the major financial sponsors. These sites were significant because of their strategic importance for the future of mobile computing in the Québec healthcare sector. Indeed, this was a pilot project that needed to go through a rigorous evaluation process to shed light on the political decision to spread this new model of homecare interventions to all homecare units in Québec. The average budget attributed to the pilot project per site amounted to Can$300,000 for a total budget of Can$2,700,000.

The sites which took part in the project were chosen so as to reflect the variety of homecare units in the Québec healthcare system. Hence, they varied in terms of number of nurses, the size of the geographic area covered, and the distribution of the patients who received homecare services. As shown in Table 1, the sample included both urban and rural programs which cover territories varying between 65 and 2,280 km^2. The number of targeted mobile computing users in these units varied from 7 to 25.

Further, one of the original characteristics of the project was the implementation of a global governance structure. This structure, which is depicted in Fig. 1,

Table 1 Profile of the homecare sites

	Site 1	Site 2	Site 3	Site 4	Site 5	Site 6	Site 7	Site 8	Site 9
Territory and population covered									
Territory covered (km^2)	1,491	66	1,500	1,400	n/d	852	2,279	1,267	830
Total number of residents	57,796	77,355	60,000	21,744	55,000	125,000	19,425	33,947	83,947
Number of residents/km^2	38.8	1,172.0	40.0	15.5	n/d	146.7	8.5	26.8	101.1
Nursing staff									
Number of nurses involved in the project	11	7	16	7	25	19	11	16	25
Total number of active patients	615	n/d	449	165	1,224	941	298	407	906
Case-load (Average numberof patients per nurse)	75–80	45	50	58	65	100	45–50	129	57
Nurses' resources from private agencies	None	Yes	None	Yes	Yes	Yes	Yes	None	Yes
Financial situation									
Establishment experiencing a budget deficit	Yes	None	None	None	Yes	Yes	None	None	None

not only had to act as a traditional steering committee but also had to ensure knowledge transfer and emulation between sites.

4.2 Mobile Technology

The SyMO^{TM} mobile technology software was intended to optimize the process used to plan and organize nursing activities in patients' homes. The mobile technology enabled patient clinical data management at multiple locations (patient's home, on the road, homecare program office or even healthcare professional's own home), both in terms of data visualization and entry. The application included a series of automated care plans, clinical assessment tools and order forms to support registered nurses in patient evaluation and treatment, visit scheduling, follow-up and case load care planning. Data sharing with other members of the care team was also possible.

The software, which was installed on a portable computer, consisted of a series of modules. It was first composed of a dictionary of nursing care plans that covered all the procedures registered nurses need to perform in response to patient health problems (e.g., assessing physical pain, weighing patients, teaching patients). For

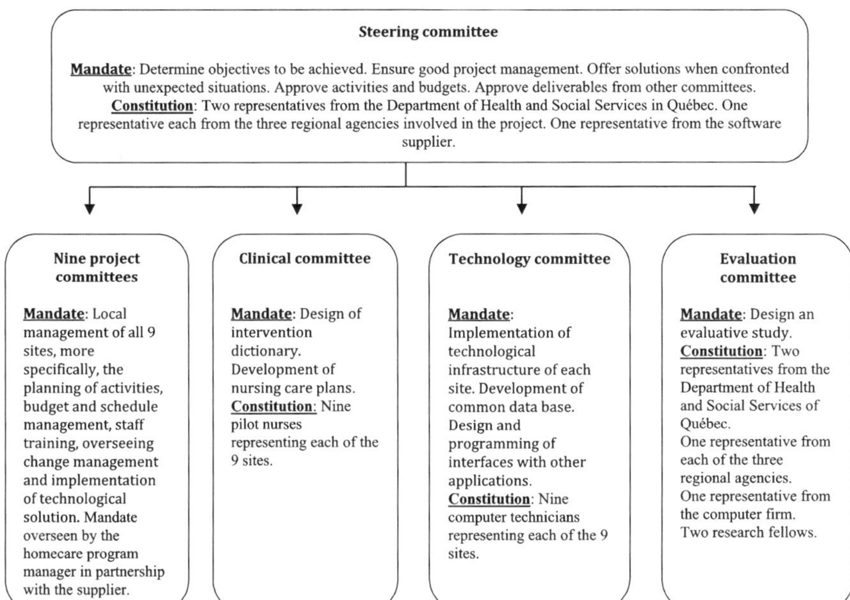

Fig. 1 Project governance structure

each intervention, the dictionary suggested a frequency (e.g., once every 3 days, once a week), the time typically required for the procedure (in minutes) and other details (e.g., use of a particular type of bandage). The version of the dictionary contained about 40 nursing care plan models, organized by system type (e.g., the pulmonary system, the digestive system). The nurse's role consisted in evaluating the health status of patients and creating the appropriate treatment plan for them. Through the Intervention Plan module, the nursed entered the list of actions to be undertaken with the patient. At the patient's home, the nurse also used the Patient Diary module, which provided a list of the interventions to be performed; it allowed her to take notes. The nurse could enter a note for each procedure in the patient's care plan. This module was aimed at enhancing both the quality and continuity of care by providing access to the full history of nursing records associated with each intervention. The future version of the mobile software will include other categories of users such as social workers, attending physicians, and other homecare professionals.

4.3 Conceptual Framework and Measures

As shown in Fig. 2, our conceptual framework is comprised of three constructs, namely, the nature and level of project risk, the risk mitigation strategy, and the extent of project success. As mentioned previously, we used a classification of risk

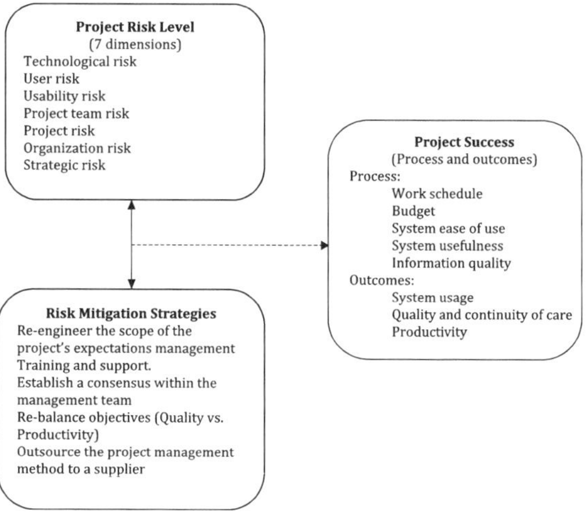

Fig. 2 Conceptual framework

factors in order to evaluate the project's nature and level of risk at all nine sites. The identification of the risk management strategies was devised in an inductive manner during semi-structured interviews with project team members and users of the new system at each site. The project risk measure as well as the success of the mobile computing project was also multidimensional in nature. This measure encompassed eight criteria. The first two criteria enabled us to evaluate the adherence to the schedule and budget of each site. These data were available in the minutes of the project steering committee meetings. The remaining six criteria were based on nurses' perceptions of the benefits offered by the new system. Three process criteria (system ease of use, system usefulness, information quality) and three result criteria (system usage, quality and continuity of care, productivity) enabled us to evaluate the nurses' perceptions. The reliability validity of all scales was assessed through the analysis of the internal consistency of each scale, that is, the extent to which the items are homogeneous. In this sense, reliability refers to the accuracy or precision of a measuring instrument. This was tested by calculating Cronbach's alpha for each criteria. Normally, it is established that a target level of minimum reliability would be set at 0.70. Scales for system ease of use (3 items, alpha = .90) and system usefulness (3 items, alpha = .90) were adapted from Venkatesh et al. [30]. Information quality (7 items, alpha = .92) was measured using an instrument from Bailey and Pearson [3]. Scale for system use (6 items, alpha = .89) was developed to meet the specific needs of this study. The scales for quality and continuity of nursing care (5 items, alpha = .86) were adapted from Sicotte et al. [27]; and the scale used to assess nurses' productivity (4 items, alpha = .87) was developed for the specific needs of this study. All measures used a 10-point ordinal scale with anchors ranging from "strongly disagree" to "strongly agree" for the items related to the process criteria, and from "very negative impact" to "very positive impact" for the items associated with the result dimensions.

4.4 Data Collection and Validity Issues

Data were primarily collected via 57 semi-structured interviews with project leaders, nurse users, and nurse pilots. The interviews were used to identify the risk factors, their intensity and the corresponding risk mitigation strategies. In addition, structured questionnaires and administrative data were used to establish the level of project success.

Data collection occurred over three periods of time. The first series of interviews was performed at the end of the requirements analysis at each site (T1), approximately 7 weeks after the kick-off meeting. The second series of interviews was conducted 2–3 months later, while the system go-live period was underway (T2). A first group of nurses was then trained. This group used the system on a regular basis during their homecare interventions. These two series of interviews were performed between September 2008 and April 2009.

The list of key sources was varied and enabled a wide understanding according to various points of view. At each site, key respondents included the head of the homecare program who acted as local project manager; a pilot nurse who was responsible for dispensing training and support for the new system; the head of the information technology department; a manager from the software supplier firm; and a minimum of three nurse users. Two research team members were present at each site and conducted the interviews. Complete confidentiality of data collected was ensured in order to restrict any links between risks identified and the identity of those who had mentioned them. Hence, everyone could express themselves freely. It enabled an in-depth understanding of the stage of implementation progress at each site.

The content of all interviews was analyzed and synthesized using a set of datasheets which described the nature and intensity of each of the 30 risk factors. Each sheet was associated with a risk factor. It referenced favorable as well as problematic elements related to a given factor, identified the intensity of risk (high, moderate, low, very low), and proposed one or several measures to limit risk. The datasheets were first completed by the research team members who had conducted the interviews. The sheets were then cross-checked by another member of the research team to ensure internal consistency as well as consistency between sites. Following this, all datasheets were submitted to the local project manager for further validation and to encourage the project team to take any action necessary to ensure project success.

Lastly, the third data collection point was associated with the evaluation of the project's success (T3). In order to estimate the success of the project at each site, we analyzed administrative data and survey data. The administrative data allowed us to assess the adherence to the schedule and budget. The survey occurred 3 months after all nursing personnel had been trained to use the new system. We asked all 137 nurse users involved in the project to complete a structured questionnaire that measured the effects of the mobile technology on their work. A total of 101 completed questionnaires were returned to the investigators, representing a 74% response rate.

4.5 Data Processing of the Risk Dimensions Scores

As we just mentioned, the content of all interviews was analyzed and synthesized using a set of datasheets which described the nature and intensity of each of the 30 risk factors composing our analytical framework. These data are presented in detail in Appendix 2. For each of the nine sites, at $T1$ and $T2$, we thus had an intensity level for each risk factor categorized according to four levels: VL = Very low risk (0 point); L = Low risk (1 point); M = Moderate risk (2 points); H = High risk (3 points). As specified in the parentheses, a number of points was associated with each level. The addition of points enabled the calculation of seven risk dimension scores corresponding to each of the seven dimensions of our analytical framework. Also, it was possible to calculate an overall risk score varying between 0 and 90 (30 risk factors multiplied by three, the maximum of the four-level scale). These dimensional and overall scores are presented in Table 2 as percentages that are the intensity scores divided by the maximum of the corresponding scale.

5 Results

5.1 Project Risk Analysis

Table 2 introduces the nature and level of risk observed at each site such as it was assessed at $T1$ and $T2$. This assessment takes the form of a global score which qualifies the degree of intensity of risks recorded at each site in terms of number of points and percentage and supplies an average for the sites as a whole. This table also shows the evolution of variations with respect to the number of risk factors and dimensions. Last, it presents the specific scores of each of the seven risk dimensions for $T1$ and $T2$ at each site. Appendix 2 details the risk analysis which enabled the computation of scores shown in Table 2.

5.2 The Average Global Risk

As shown in Table 2, the average global risk scores reached a mean level of 32 over a scale of 90 points for an average risk percentage of 36% (that is 32—the overall risk level—divided by 90—the possible maximum overall risk level). The variation of global risk scores, by site, varied from 29 to 46%. Such a risk level could be qualified as moderately high. Importantly, the global intensity risk level decreased between $T1$ and $T2$ at all sites. Scores observed at $T1$ were indeed

Table 2 Cross-case risk analysis

Overall risk[a]	Risk intensity																		
	Site 1		Site 2		Site 3		Site 4		Site 5		Site 6		Site 7		Site 8		Site 9		Mean
	T1	T2	T1	T2	T1	T2	T1	T2	T1	T2	T1	T2	T1	T2	T1	T2	T1	T2	
Overall risk score [0–90]	32	28	41	35	37	30	33	29	32	30	34	31	29	27	40	33	33	26	32
	36%[b]	31%	46%	39%	41%	33%	37%	32%	36%	33%	38%	34%	32%	30%	44%	37%	37%	29%	36%
Variation between T1 and T2	−4		−6		−7		−4		−2		−3		−2		−7		−7		−4.7
Number of dimensions with at least one moderate risk factor	5	2	5	5	5	2	4	2	4	2	4	3	4	3	5	5	4	1	3.6
Variation between T1 and T2	−3		0		−3		−2		−2		−1		−1		0		−3		−1.7
Technological (5 Risk factors/Score [0–15])	20%[c]	20%	20%	20%	20%	20%	20%	20%	20%	20%	20%	27%	20%	20%	20%	20%	20%	20%	20%
Users (5 Risk factors/Score [0-15])	33%[d]	27%	53%	40%	60%	27%	47%	27%	47%	27%	53%	33%	40%	27%	66%	40%	47%	27%	39%
Usability (3 Risk factors/Score [0–9])	56%[d]	78%	78%	44%	56%	56%	66%	66%	66%	66%	66%	66%	44%	44%	66%	66%	56%	33%	60%
Project team (4 Risk factors/Score [0–12])	42%[d]	33%	50%	42%	42%	33%	33%	33%	33%	33%	33%	33%	33%	33%	50%	50%	33%	33%	36%
Project (6 Risk factors/Score [0–18])	33%[d]	28%	50%	50%	44%	50%	33%	39%	33%	44%	33%	33%	33%	39%	39%	33%	44%	39%	39%
Organization (3 Risk factors/Score [0–9])	56%[d]	33%	66%	66%	56%	33%	44%	33%	44%	33%	44%	33%	56%	44%	66%	44%	44%	33%	46%
Strategic / Political / Legal (4 Risk factors/Score [0–12])	17%[d]	17%	17%	17%	17%	17%	17%	17%	17%	17%	17%	17%	17%	17%	17%	17%	17%	17%	17%

[a] Overall risk score was composed of 30 risk factors, each varying between 0 and 3 points according to the risk level [VL = Very low risk (0 point); L = Low risk (1 point); M = Moderate risk (2 points); H = High risk (3 points)]. The detailed analysis appears in Appendix 2

[b] The risk intensity percentage is calculated by taking the risk intensity score divided by the maximum of the overall risk score scale (90). For instance, 36% is 32—the overall risk level—divided by 90—the possible maximum overall risk level

[c] The Technological risk intensity percentage is calculated by taking the Technological risk intensity score divided by the maximum of the Technological risk score scale (15). The detailed analysis enabling the calculation of the Technological risk score appears in Appendix 2

[d] The percentage of this risk dimension score is calculated as the technological risk intensity percentage (see #c)

systematically higher than at *T*2. The first evaluations varied from 32 to 46%, while evaluations recorded at *T*2 varied from 29 to 39%. The largest reduction of risk reached a magnitude of 8% while the lowest reduction of risk was 2%. With respect to the count of risk factors, this decrease of intensity entailed a decrease ranging from two to seven risk factors.

5.3 The Dispersion of Risks

In order to fully evaluate the project risk, it is also useful to analyze the dispersion of risks among the seven dimensions which make up the framework. The higher the risk dimension, the more difficult the situation is, as the project management team must use various mitigating approaches to try and reduce risk. Table 2 indicates that, at *T*1, risks encountered at four sites were dispersed among five of the seven dimensions while risks observed at the remaining five sites were associated with four of the seven dimensions. At *T*2, all but two sites were able to reduce the spread of risk factors. Three of the sites were even able to reduce their dispersion factor by three dimensions and, one site (site #9) was able to concentrate its risk factors within a single dimension.

5.4 The Political Risk

We also analyzed the nature of risk dimensions observed in all sites. As shown in Table 2, some risk dimensions remained minor issues while others became more important throughout the project. The political risk was the dimension with the least impact at all sites. This dimension obtained the lowest scores (average intensity level = 17%) and scores associated with this dimension remained consistent from *T*1 to *T*2 for all sites. From a political perspective, all stakeholders within the Québec Department of Health, the three regional agencies and the nine homecare units quickly recognized the importance of trying to provide better support to nurses in homecare work, more specifically with respect to a context where the shortage of labor is acute. Therefore, all parties agreed on the project vision and objectives.

5.5 The Technological Risk

Similar findings were recorded with respect to technological risk. Indeed, this risk dimension remained relatively low (average intensity level = 20%) from *T*1 to *T*2. From a technological viewpoint, the new system was relatively mature. The system had previously been tested in the same type of organization and had consequently been improved so as to supply well adjusted homecare plans. The system's response time was also adequate. A reliable and high performing computer network was already in place at all the sites before the new technology implementation. At one site (site #6), technology risk was deemed slightly higher than at others (average intensity level = 27%); this was due to an external factor. In this specific case, a local computer network problem had undermined the response time performance of the new mobile system during the $T2$ data collection period.

5.6 The Usability Risk

The remaining five risk dimensions registered higher intensity levels as well as wider variations in time and across sites. For one thing, the highest risk scores were associated with the Usability risk dimension (average intensity level = 60%). The three risk factors which make up this dimension had a major impact on the high degree of risk recorded. First, the usability of the new system presented a major challenge. The complexity of the software was mostly connected to the exhaustive degree of the clinical content (40 nursing care plans) and the learning of the various navigation pathways required to suitably document a patient's file. The perceived usability of the new system also contributed to risk intensity. Some confusion was indeed apparent among the nurses with respect to the main underlying reason for introducing a new system within their unit, that is, the improvement of care quality in opposition to an increase of nursing productivity. As well, managers in charge of the project had suggested that the new system would eliminate the duplication of manual data entry between the various existing information systems. In order to reach this objective, various software interfaces had to be created to ensure the exchange of data between the new system and the existing clinical-administrative software applications of the various sites (e.g., patient admissions, patient treatment plans). However, the scope of work required precluded the development of these interfaces during the project. Finally, the lack of downstream and upstream processes between the new system and the execution of homecare visits constituted one of the major project risk factors. There were some efforts undertaken towards process harmonization, but they remained limited to homecare services. Therefore, this transformation did not reach the support services, such as admissions, archiving and the medical supply, which interact with homecare services on a regular basis. Overall, the intensity of the risk associated with the usability dimension remained stable or decreased slightly between $T1$ and $T2$ at all the sites, with the exception of one site (site #1) where a major increase was recorded.

5.7 The Organization Risk

Next, two risk factors contributed to the intensity of the Organization risk dimension (average intensity level = 46%). The first factor was the organizational instability which was common in the great majority of sites. It was often mentioned, during interviews, that various changes in practices, structures, and upper management were occurring during the implementation of the new system which had a major effect on everyone, along with a sense of weariness. Secondly, the lack of support from upper management turned out to be a significant negative factor at two of the sites (sites #2 and #8). It should be noted that the project was rapidly implemented on the initiative of regional agencies and that various local upper management levels took quite a while to become involved in the project. The project was perceived as a technological change by many sites. The scope of organizational change had been greatly underestimated. This lack of involvement by the administration hindered the proper functioning, particularly at $T1$.

5.8 The Project Team, Users and Project Risks

Lastly, data from Table 2 indicate that the remaining three risk dimensions reached similar levels (36% for Project Team risk dimension and 39% for both the Users and Project risk dimensions). At most of the sites, the risk intensity associated with these three dimensions decreased between $T1$ and $T2$. However, there are certain sites where the risk remained stable over time, more specifically in relation to the Usability and Project Team risk dimensions. Finally, the risk intensity associated with the Project risk dimension also increased slightly between $T1$ and $T2$ for three of the nine sites (sites #4, 5 and 7).

In short, the detailed analysis of risk by dimension highlighted the fact that some risk dimensions were particularly sensitive (Usability and Organization) and that some sites met with much greater difficulty than others. In the next section, we will assess the project's success level for each site. Then, we will review which mitigating approaches were implemented to limit the risks associated with the implementation of the mobile solution. This analysis will help us identify the critical success factors which represent efficient management strategies for reducing risk, and fostering successful technology implementation.

5.9 The Extent of Project Success

As mentioned earlier, the success of the mobile computing project was evaluated using five implementation (process) criteria and three benefit (outcomes) criteria. Table 3 introduces the results computed at each of the nine sites. The first process criterion was aimed at measuring the adherence to the budget established at the outset of the project. The measure of success relied on reaching a target of $\pm 5\%$ with respect to the initial budget. As shown in Table 3, all sites met this criterion. The second criterion, adherence to the project deadline, was evaluated in much the same manner. Five sites encountered a 2 week delay (8% in time duration), while the maximum delay for the two other sites was 4 weeks (15%). The main cause of these delays is attributable to summer vacations which had a bigger impact than originally foreseen. The remaining six success criteria were based on the opinions of the nurses involved in the project. Overall, results associated with these criteria

Table 3 Assessment of project success

	Site 1	Site 2	Site 3	Site 4	Site 5	Site 6	Site 7	Site 8	Site 9	Overall mean
Process criteria										
Project realized within budget	Yes	Yes	Yes	Yes	Yes	Yes	Yes	Yes	Yes	Yes
System delivered on schedule	2 week delay	2 week delay	1 month delay	On time	1 month delay	3 week delay	2 week delay	2 week delay	2 week delay	2.3 weeks
Quality of information system										
Ease of use	8.1	8.5	7.5	6.9	7.7	7.2	8.4	7.4	7.3	7.7
Usefulness	8.3	8.3	7.7	6.6	7.4	7.0	8.3	6.8	6.8	7.5
Information quality	8.9	8.7	8.0	8.1	8.1	7.8	8.7	7.9	8.1	8.3
Outcomes criteria										
Level of system use sophistication	8.2	6.7	7.5	7.0	6.7	6.9	7.7	7.7	7.1	7.3
Perceived benefits										
Quality and continuity of care	8.6	8.4	7.6	7.2	7.3	7.4	8.7	7.0	6.4	7.6
Staff productivity	8.1	7.5	7.2	7.5	6.0	6.5	7.8	6.6	6.6	7.1

were positive. The average scores recorded for all the sites varied from 7.1 (improved nurse productivity) to 8.3 (improved quality of clinical information) on a scale of 10.

In short, 3 months after the system go-live at each site, the whole project can be considered successful. For one thing, the mobile technology was deployed on time and within budget. Next, the nurse users had adopted the mobile application and we were told that it was still in use at all sites 1 year after deployment. Importantly, nurses perceived that the system had positive effects on the quality and continuity of homecare services and their own level of productivity.

5.10 Mitigation Risk Measures

In order to better understand how the sites under study reached their observed level of success despite the risks they encountered, we will now analyze the mitigating measures which were implemented. It is important to note that all nine sites put their greatest efforts towards those risk factors that were most problematic. We, therefore, observed a close alignment between the intensity of efforts pertaining to mitigating management and the intensity of risks involved.

5.11 Clarifying the Vision

Among the most common mitigating approaches, communication efforts aiming to clarify the project scope and objectives required a great deal of energy from the project managers at most sites. With a view to better managing expectations, these efforts were aimed at reducing the most prevalent risk dimension, namely, Usability risk (average intensity level $= 60\%$). The objective was to help nurses perceive the new system not as a technological tool, but rather as a clinical tool that would help in significantly improving the quality and continuity of care offered to patients. Further, substantial efforts were directed towards training and support to ensure the early development of positive attitudes towards the new system. Training and support were dispensed, from the onset of the project, by a pilot nurse who had been selected among nurses involved at each site. Each of these pilot nurses was also actively involved in the clinical committee meetings (Fig. 1) whose primary mandate was to develop the data base's clinical content (40 care plans), the data collecting forms, and the format for reports generated by the system.

5.12 Aligning the New System and Local Work Practices

Despite the measures specified previously, the intensity of risks associated with the Usability risk dimension remained relatively high for most sites because of the lack of alignment between the new system and local work practices. As mentioned previously, very little effort had been devoted to the harmonization of the new system with respect to the downstream and upstream processes of homecare visits (planning of visits, management of medical supplies, requests to the archives department). Furthermore, the objective associated with the elimination of duplication of manual data capture, which was emphasized during the kick-off meeting, could not be met because of the software package's lack of interoperability with the existing clinical-administrative applications and delays associated with the development of system interfaces. So the initial expectations with respect to the potential benefits of the new system were not managed appropriately. When the new system was "sold" to the nurses during the kick-off meeting, it was somehow introduced as a nearly perfect product that would solve all their problems. This proved to be an inadequate approach. Communication efforts, therefore, became necessary so as to re-formulate and lower the original messages while explaining that developments were ongoing to, on one hand, ensure the interoperability of the software package with that of the existing computer applications as well as harmonize the software application with that of lateral processes.

5.13 Clarifying users' Expectations

The ambiguity surrounding the benefits associated with the use of the mobile application also affected nurses' morale. This had a direct effect on the level of resistance to change, which is associated with the User risk dimension (average intensity level $= 39\%$). Indeed, many questions were raised by nurses with respect to the effects of the system on their nursing practices and work routines, more specifically during $T1$. Some nurses feared the new system was introduced for the sole purpose of increasing the number of home visits per work shift. Efforts aimed at clarifying the aforementioned expectations helped reduce the intensity of the User risk between $T1$ and $T2$ (see Table 2).

5.14 Counterbalancing the Project Objectives

Regarding the Organization risk dimension (average intensity level $= 46\%$), it ensued from the interviews with the heads of the homecare programs that many weeks had elapsed after the official project launch before they and the upper management team of each unit realized that the introduction of the new system was not only a technological initiative but a major project which required major organizational transformations involving changes at various levels (roles and responsibilities of each person, structures, processes, work habits, organizational culture, etc.). This erroneous conception explains, at least in part, why process reengineering efforts took so long to be implemented in the great majority of the sites. In fact, it is the risk associated with the Usability and User dimensions which sounded the alarm. Once this was acknowledged, all the sites decided to emphasize the benefits associated with the quality and continuity of care and thus to capitalize on the fact that the new system was a clinical tool which had been developed by and for nurses. As for the objective associated with the increase of the nurses' productivity, it was relegated to a medium- to long-term goal. This strategy which consisted in prioritizing quality objectives and deferring productivity objectives was implemented at most sites. Despite the Québec Department of Health and regional agencies' keen interest in making the financial investment profitable by increasing the nurses' productivity, upper management in each unit, along with the head of the homecare program, decided to first focus on the quality and continuity of care in order to lessen resistance to the mobile computing project and win the support of the nursing staff for system deployment, which is what was accomplished.

5.15 *The Importance of External Support*

With respect to the Project risk dimension (average intensity level = 39%), the continued support from the software supplier must be underlined and, more specifically, that of the supplier's project managers who meticulously and uniformly applied a rigorous project management methodology at every site, a mandate which had been entrusted to them at the start of the project. This helped keep the project on target both in regards to budget as well as schedule.

Lastly, the risk associated with the Project Team risk dimension (average intensity level = 36%) was also reduced at every site from $T1$ to $T2$. Project teams, which consisted of people with complementary expertise (clinical, management, technology, archives), received efficient support from the supplier's project managers throughout the undertaking. Only one site (site #8) encountered serious problems; they were attributable to the lack of experience of an interim program manager.

6 Discussion

The objective of this study was to better understand the phenomenon surrounding the implementation of mobile technology within the home care context. As such, the research pursued two main goals. First, it tried to identify factors which could affect the deployment of the technology. To this end, a risk analysis model was used to enable the identification of a vast range of risks that could affect the success of such projects. Furthermore and within the framework of a risk management contingent approach, the research tried to identify which mitigating strategies would likely limit the risks involved and foster project success.

A first main finding allowed us to bring to light the multiplicity and variability of problematic issues associated with risks encountered in this type of project. It was clear from our findings that risks involved do not have the same level of intensity. Technological risk which, for many, should be a major risk with respect to projects relying on the use of technological innovation, turned out to be relatively low at all sites. Cross analysis of all nine cases clearly highlighted the critical importance of other types of risk, notably, Usability, User and Organization. These results are in keeping with the few studies which analyzed the adoption of mobile technologies by health professionals. The expected usefulness and ease of use—which are in line with the Usability risks—are indeed critical factors which were identified in one of the studies [35]. A second study, which analyzed the attitudes of health professionals with respect to using mobile technology in a real healthcare context, also identified the major role of the usefulness factor [37]. Lastly, it is interesting to highlight the fact that our findings pertaining to risk factor intensity are also aligned with the opinions of experts who took part in the Delphi study which is at the root of the analysis grid used in the present research project [21]. These experts had also relegated the technological risk factor to last place and prioritized the importance of risks associated with Project, Organization and Usability dimensions (Appendix 2 shows the ranking that these experts gave to each of the 30 risk factors).

Another interesting finding is the presence of a strong interdependency between risk dimensions. Indeed, analyzed data highlights the link which exists between the risk factors inasmuch as the levels of intensity of some risks have a ripple effect on others. As such, the Usability and Organization risks are closely intertwined at all sites. This finding is in line with results from another study on CIS implementation which adopted a similar taxonomy [26]. This study highlighted the fact that risk factors were closely intertwined and that systematic ripple effects from one risk factor to another were frequent.

A third main finding highlighted the importance of a contingent risk management strategy. In other words, prioritizing management efforts around more intense and threatening risks was an effective strategy which fostered a positive outcome. As such, our findings introduce various interesting lessons for the management of this type of project. Among the major lessons, we must first mention the strategic importance of suitably managing user expectations. Then, we must also mention two strategies which were particularly useful in small organizations such as the ones under study. Management teams from small health organizations are often overworked and rarely have suitable competencies in project management. All the sites under study benefited from significant outside support which was supplied in all cases. First, the concerted efforts from the application supplier and the steering committee had a major positive influence on the rigorous management method used and therefore also on the ensuing level of success. Secondly, the high visibility associated with the project assessment and the inherent comparisons between sites played a major role in terms of the attention and efforts which were exerted locally by management teams and program managers alike with respect to implementation. Lastly, we must recognize that there is a limit to be observed with respect to the quantity and scope of organizational changes which can be undertaken at the same time, especially in small organizations. Several organizations under study were hit hard in this regard. In this case, a high priority was granted to the mobile computing project, mostly because of the two measures which we just described. In common occurrences of solely local change management, it is more than likely that these projects would not have attracted the same sense of urgency to act and we would surely have encountered a greater number of failures.

Before concluding, it is important to recognize the limitations of this study. First, even though we used a multiple-case analysis, it is possible that the specificity of cases under study might restrict the generalization of our findings. However, we think that the generalization of our findings could be broadly applied because risk factors identified are typical of the organizational change initiatives seen in the broader management literature [2, 9, 16, 25]. Moreover, it is evident that the status of pilot projects and the presence of an evaluation research had a significant effect on the level of attention and effort of the project managers. Without undermining the importance of this factor, we believe the lesson to be learned from this is that high visibility and external supports are critical to achieving success. The challenge then is to ensure the implementation of these success-fostering mechanisms. As such, the governance structure implemented in this project was a major asset and could become a source of inspiration for similar projects. Lastly, we must recognize that it could very well be more difficult to reproduce the same results in larger organizations. The small number of users for each site enabled a customized training strategy, communications and supervisory activities. This situation would certainly be more difficult to reproduce in larger health organizations. Finally, the project under study entailed a specific type of mobile computing application which was devised for nurses only. It would, therefore, be essential to conduct similar studies to confirm and generalize our findings.

7 Conclusion

The increase and improvement of home care is perceived as a means of dispensing quality care to an ageing population suffering from a growing number of chronic illnesses. While information technology such as mobile computing offers interesting innovative solutions, we must remember that the implementation of such technologies remains a major challenge especially with respect to small health organizations where these technologies are most often implemented. Major efforts must be expended on planning and supporting these projects. We hope our findings will help inspire future projects.

Acknowledgments The authors would like to thank Mr. Daniel Caron, Paul-Yvon Forest and Richard Labbé for their contribution during the data collection phase. They would also like to thank all the personnel from the nine sites who generously accepted to take part in this study. Finally, the Québec Department of Health and the participating regional agencies are gratefully acknowledged for their financial support.

A.1 8   Appendix

Appendix 1 CIS project risk framework

Risk Dimensions	Risk Factors
Technological	Introduction of a new technology
	Complex/unreliable technical infrastructure or network
	Complex software solution
	Complex/incompatible hardware
	Poor software performance
Users	Unrealistic expectations
	Overall resistance to change
	Lack of cooperation/commitment from users
	Poor computer skills
	Prior negative experiences with CIS projects
Usability	Poor perceived system ease of use
	Poor perceived system usefulness
	Misalignment of system with local practices and processes
Project Team	Changes to membership on the project team
	Poor project leadership
	Lack of required knowledge or skills
	Lack of clear role definitions
	Negative attitude of project team members
Project	Large and complex project
	Project ambiguity
	Changes to requirements
	Insufficient resources
	Lack of a project champion
	Lack of a formal project management methodology
Organization/Environment	Lack of commitment from upper management
	Organizational instability
	Lack of local personnel knowledgeable in IT
	Legal and ethical constraints
Strategic/Political	Misalignment of actors' and partners' objectives and stakes
	Political games/conflicts
	Unreliable external partners

Appendix 2 Detailed risk analyses

Risk Dimensions	Risk Factors	Rank[a]	Site 1		Site 2		Site 3		Site 4		Site 5		Site 6		Site 7		Site 8		Site 9	
			T1	T2	T1	T2	T1	T2	T1	T2	T1	T2	T1	T2	T1	T2	T1	T2	T1	T2
Technological	Introduction of a new technology	22	L	L	L	L	L	L	L	L	L	L	L	L	L	L	L	L	L	L
	Complex/unreliable technical infrastructure or network	20	L	L	L	L	L	L	L	L	L	L	L	L	L	L	L	L	L	L
	Complex software solution	18	VL	VL	VL	VL	VL	VL	VL	VL	VL	VL	VL	VL	VL	VL	VL	VL	VL	VL
	Complex/incompatible hardware	21	VL	VL	VL	VL	VL	VL	VL	VL	VL	VL	VL	VL	VL	VL	VL	VL	VL	VL
	Poor software performance	11	L	L	L	L	L	L	L	L	L	L	L	M	L	L	L	L	L	L
Users	Unrealistic expectations	13	M	L	M	L	H	L	M	L	M	L	M	M	M	L	M	L	M	L
	Overall resistance to change	–	L	L	M	M	M	L	M	L	M	L	M	L	L	L	H	M	M	L
	Lack of cooperation/commitment to change	–	L	L	M	M	M	L	L	L	L	L	M	L	L	L	H	M	L	L
	Poor computer skills	23	L	L	M	L	M	L	M	L	M	L	M	L	M	L	M	L	M	L
	Prior negative experiences with IT projects	–	VL	VL	VL	VL	VL	VL	VL	VL	VL	VL	VL	VL	VL	VL	VL	VL	VL	VL
Usability	Poor perceived system ease of use	14	L	M	M	L	M	M	M	M	M	M	M	L	L	L	M	M	M	L
	Poor perceived system usefulness	3	M	M	M	L	L	L	M	M	M	M	M	M	L	L	M	M	L	L
	Misalignment of system with local processes	5	M	H	H	M	M	M	M	M	M	M	M	H	M	M	M	M	M	L
Project team	High turnover among project team members	8	M	L	L	L	M	L	L	L	L	L	L	L	L	L	L	M	L	L
	Lack of required knowledge or skills	7	L	L	M	M	L	L	L	L	L	L	L	L	L	L	L	L	L	L
	Lack of clear role definitions	–	L	L	M	L	L	L	L	L	L	L	L	L	L	L	L	L	L	L
	Negative attitudes of project team members	12	L	L	L	L	L	L	L	L	L	L	L	L	L	L	H	M	L	L

(continued)

Appendix 2 (continued)

Risk Dimensions	Risk Factors	Rank[a]	Site 1 T1	Site 1 T2	Site 2 T1	Site 2 T2	Site 3 T1	Site 3 T2	Site 4 T1	Site 4 T2	Site 5 T1	Site 5 T2	Site 6 T1	Site 6 T2	Site 7 T1	Site 7 T2	Site 8 T1	Site 8 T2	Site 9 T1	Site 9 T2
Project	Large and complex project	16	L	L	L	M	L	M	L	M	L	M	L	M	L	M	L	M	L	M
	Project ambiguity	4	H	M	H	M	H	H	M	M	M	M	M	M	M	M	M	M	H	M
	Changes to system requirements	–	L	L	L	L	L	L	L	L	L	L	L	L	L	L	L	L	L	L
	Insufficient resources	10	L	L	H	H	M	M	L	L	L	M	M	L	L	L	H	L	M	L
	Lack of a champion	1	VL	VL	L	L	L	L	L	L	L	L	VL	VL	L	L	VL	VL	L	L
	Lack of a formal project management methodology	–	VL	VL	VL	VL	VL	VL	VL	VL	VL	VL	VL	VL	VL	VL	VL	VL	VL	VL
Organization	Lack of commitment from upper management	2	M	L	H	M	L	L	L	L	L	L	L	L	L	L	M	L	L	L
	Organizational instability	9	M	L	M	H	H	L	M	L	M	L	M	L	M	L	H	M	M	L
	Lack of support/expertise from IT department	19	L	L	L	L	L	L	L	L	L	L	L	L	M	M	L	L	L	L
Strategic/ Political/ Legal	Legal and ethical constraints	17	VL	VL	VL	VL	VL	VL	VL	VL	VL	VL	VL	VL	VL	VL	VL	VL	VL	VL
	Misalignment of actors' and partners' objectives	–	L	L	L	L	L	L	L	L	L	L	L	L	L	L	L	L	L	L
	Political games/conflicts	6	L	L	L	L	L	L	L	L	L	L	L	L	L	L	L	L	L	L
	Unreliable external partners	15	VL	VL	VL	VL	VL	VL	VL	VL	VL	VL	VL	VL	VL	VL	VL	VL	VL	VL

[a] Final ranking in Paré et al. [20]. Items with no ranking number did not appear in the final list

Legend: VL = Very low risk (0 point); L = Low risk (1 point); M = Moderate risk (2 points); H = High risk (3 points)

References

1. Archer N. Is return on investment a valid criterion for investing in mobile healthcare. International conference on the management of mobile business. Toronto canada; 2007.
2. Baccarini D, Salm G, Love ED. Management of risks in information technology projects. Ind Manag Data Syst. 2004;104(3/4):286–95.
3. Bailey JE, Pearson SW. Development of a tool for measuring and analyzing computer user satisfaction. Manag Sci. 1983;29(5):530–45.
4. Baraldi S, Memmola M. How healthcare organisations actually use the internet's virtual space: a field study. Int J Healthcare Technol Manag. 2006;7(3/4):187–207.
5. Berg M. Patient care information systems and health care work: a socio-technical approach. Int J Med Inform. 1999;55(1):87–101.
6. Dang S, Dimmick S, Kelkar G. Evaluating the evidence base for the use of home tele-health remote monitoring in elderly with heart failure. J Telemed e-Health. 2009;1(9):783–96.
7. DelliFraine JL, Dansky KH. Home-based tele-health: a review and meta-analysis. J Telemed Telecare. 2008;14(2):62–6.
8. Durrani H, Khoja S. A systematic review of the use of tele-health in Asian countries. J Telemed Telecare. 2009;15(4):175–81.
9. Gibson CF. IT-enabled business change: an approach to understanding and managing risk. MIS Q Executive. 2003;2(2):104–15.
10. Goodhue DL, Thompson RL. Task–technology fit and individual performance. MIS Quarterly. 1995;19(2):213–36.
11. Hameed K. The application of mobile computing and technology to health care services. Telematics Inform. 2003;20(2):99–106.
12. Heeks R. Health information systems: Failure, success and improvisation. Int J Med Inform. 2006;75:125–37.
13. Hong HS, Kim IK, Lee SH, Kim HS. Adoption of PDA-based home hospice care system for cancer patients. Comp, Inform, Nurs. 2009;27(6):365–71.
14. Kairy D, Lehoux P, Vincent C, Visintin M. A systematic review of clinical outcomes, clinical processes, healthcare utilization and costs associated with telerehabilitation. Disabil Rehabil. 2009;31(6):427–47.
15. Lapointe L, Rivard S. A triple take on information system implementation. Organ Sci. 2007;18(1):89–107.
16. Lorenzi NM, Riley RT. Organizational aspects of health informatics: Managing technological change. New York: Springer Verlag; 1995.
17. May C, Finch T, Mair F, Mort M. Towards a wireless patient: Chronic illness, scarce care and technological innovation in the United Kingdom. Soc Sci Med. 2005;61:1485–94.
18. Nicolini D. The work to make telemedicine work: a social and articulate view. Soc Sci Med. 2006;62:2754–67.
19. OECD (Organization for Economic Co-operation and Development). Healthcare expenditure: a future in question (cited 2010 May 15). Available from: http://www.oecdobserver.org/news/fullstory.php/aid/556/Healthcare_expenditure_:_a_future_in_question.html.
20. Paré G, Jaana M, Sicotte C. Systematic review of home tele-monitoring for chronic diseases: the evidence base. J Am Med Inform Assoc. 2007;14(3):269–77.
21. Paré G, Sicotte C, Jaana M, Girouard D. Prioritizing the risk factors influencing the success of clinical information system projects: a delphi study in Canada. Met Inform Med. 2008;47(3):251–9.
22. Paré G, Sicotte C, Chekli M, Jaana M, DeBlois C, Bouchard M. A pre-post evaluation of a tele-homecare program in oncology and palliative care. Telemed e-Health. 2009;15(2):154–9.
23. Paré G, Moqadem K, Pineau G, St-Hilaire C. Clinical effectiveness of home tele-monitoring programs in the context of diabetes, asthma, heart failure and hypertension: a systematic review. J Med Internet Res. 2010;15(2):e21.

24. Polisena J, Tran K, Cimon K, Hutton B, McGill S, Palmer K, Scott RE. Home tele-health for congestive heart failure: a systematic review and meta-analysis. J Telemed Telecare. 2010;16(2):68–76.
25. Sherer SA, Alter S. Information system risks and risk factors. Commun AIS. 2004;14(1):29–64.
26. Sicotte C, Paré G. Success in health information exchange projects: Solving the implementation puzzle. Soc Sci Med. 2010;70:1159–65.
27. Sicotte C, Paré G, Moreault MP, Lemay A, Valiquette L, Barkun J. Replacing an inpatient electronic medical record: Lessons learned from user satisfaction with the previous system. Met Inform Med. 2009;48(1):92–100.
28. Stefanelli M. The role of methodologies to improve efficiency and effectiveness of care delivery processes for the year 2013. Int J Med Inform. 2002;66(1–3):39–44.
29. Tsiknakis M, Kouroubali A. Organizational factors affecting successful adoption of innovative eHealth services: a case study employing the FITT framework. Int J Med Inform. 2009;78:39–52.
30. Venkatesh V, Morris MG, Davis GB, Davis FD. User acceptance of information technology: Toward a unified view. MIS Q. 2003;27(3):425–78.
31. Vital Wave Consulting. Health for development—mobile communications for healthcare in the developing world 2008 (cited 2010 Aug 2). Available from http://www.vodafone.com/etc./medialib/foundation_imagery/ mhealth_brochure.Par.47902.File.tmp/unf_mhealth_for_development_brochure.pdf.
32. WHO. The World Health Report. Primary health care: Now more than ever. World Health Organization 2008 (cited 2010 May 28). Available from http://www.who.int/whr/ en/index.html.
33. WHO. The solid facts: Home care in Europe. World Health Organization 2009 (cited 2010 May 15). Available from http://www.euro.who.int/__data/assets/pdf_file/0005/96467/ E91884.pdf.
34. Wootton R, Dimmick SL, Kvedar JC. Home Telehealth: Connecting care within the community. London: Royal Soc Med Press: 2006.
35. Wu JH, Wang SC, Lin LM. Mobile computing acceptance factors in the healthcare industry: a structural equation model. Int J Med Inform. 2007;76:66–77.
36. Yuan Y, Archer N, Connelly CE, Zheng W. Identifying the ideal fit between mobile work and mobile work support. Inform Manag. 2010;47:125–37.
37. Zhang H, Cocosila M, Archer N. Factors of adoption of mobile information technology by homecare nurses: a technology acceptance model approach. Comp, Inform, Nurs. 2010;28(1):49–56.

AAL+: Continuous Institutional and Home Care Through Wireless Biosignal Monitoring Systems

Hugo Silva, Susana Palma and Hugo Gamboa

Abstract This chapter describes the research and development of AAL+, a new tool for continuous short-to-medium and long range patient monitoring. The system has two versions, each targeted at a different environment and at subjects with different needs: (a) *AAL+ Institutional*, for patients that live in healthcare institutions such as assisted living facilities, with delicate needs in terms of medical assistance and monitoring; and (b) *AAL+ Home*, for individuals that live in their homes, maintaining some independence and physical capabilities. In the next sections we describe the particular characteristics of each version as well as the development, test and deployment scenarios, in close collaboration with partners from the clinical field and end-users. Currently, the system is in a late prototype stage and was tested in a real environment at two healthcare institutions: an assisted living residence and a public hospital Users' reactions show that this system brings advantages which extend to institutions, caregivers and end-users, and translate into faster assistance, higher efficiency of the services and new intervention models.

Keywords Ambient Assited Living · Remote and Continuous Monitoring · Biosignals · Signal processing · Sensing

H. Silva (✉) · S. Palma · H. Gamboa
PLUX Engenharia de Biosensores, Lisbon, Portugal
e-mail: hsilva@plux.info

H. Silva
Instituto de Telecomunicações (IT), Lisbon, Portugal

H. Gamboa
Physics Department, FCT-UNL, Caparica, Portugal

Commun Med Care Compunetics (2011) 3: 115–142
DOI: 10.1007/8754_2011_25
© Springer-Verlag Berlin Heidelberg 2011
Published Online: 30 April 2011

1 Introduction

1.1 Aging in the Developed World

Population aging is nowadays growing to a worldwide concern. In the U.S. alone, 2008 projections indicated a 13% population share for senior citizens aged over 65 years in 2010; [1] current projections now show that by 2050 this number will have grown above 20%. For the EU countries there is a similar forecast. A recent OECD report revealed that the ratio between citizens aged over 65 and the total population was reaching 15% in 2010 and it is expected to grow above 25% until 2050 (Fig. 1) [2]. According to statistics from the Eurostat, [3] whereas in 2008, within the EU, there were four people of working age (15–64 years old) for every person aged over 65, in 2060, the ratio is expected to be 2–1.

With this generalized trend, critical issues such as providing a good quality of life, wellness and efficient healthcare services for senior citizens are rapidly arising and making way for the development of novel, efficient and cost-effective technologies. These issues, together with the higher education levels within this aged population and the widespread awareness and use of technologies in their daily lives are creating a fast growing demand for innovation in healthcare and assistive technological products, suitable for self-management at home and remote monitoring. The demand is emerging not only from individual users and their families, but also from healthcare institutions, as those technologies will help reduce healthcare delivery costs and increase the time available to accept new referrals. Furthermore, they enable caregivers to provide a faster response and better quality of care for the patients [4].

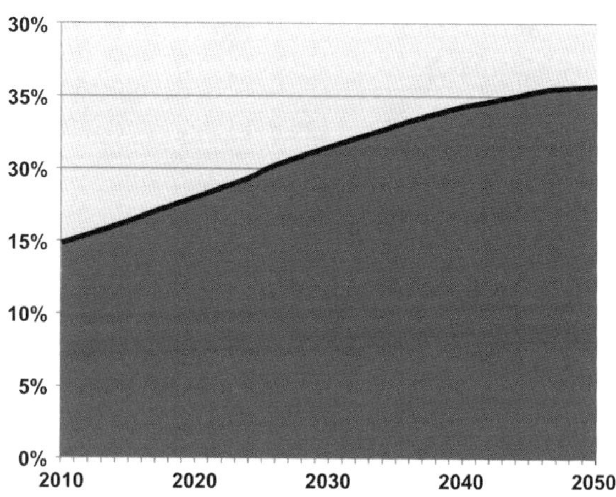

Fig. 1 Expected evolution of the ratio between citizens over 65 years and the total population within the OECD countries between 2010 and 2050

In this chapter we describe the development of devices and technologies for Ambient Assisted Living. We will focus on AAL+, a project for Ambient Assisted Living (AAL) that was born and is growing inside a startup company, although collaboration with external institutions is fostered and has already been established, namely for field tests and validation.

1.2 Ambient Assisted Living

Pervasive healthcare technologies, such as automated wearable sensing devices, are invaluable tools for regular and unobtrusive monitoring of multiple population groups. One such group is elderly people, who face specific risks related with their natural condition. Examples of these risks are involuntary falls, arrhythmia or dementia [5]. Other individuals can also benefit from pervasive healthcare technologies, namely patients with conditions such as hypertension, diabetes, heart failure and coronary heart disease, stroke, chronic pain, chronic obstructive pulmonary disease, wounds, depression and mental health problems, dementia or palliative care.

The general objective of AAL+ is to improve the efficiency, wellness, quality of care and assistance delivered to each individual, in particular elderly people, dementia and chronic patients, under an AAL framework, which is understood as follows [5, 6]:

- to extend the time people can live in their preferred environment by increasing their autonomy, self-confidence and mobility;
- to support on maintaining health and functional capability of the elderly individuals;
- to promote a better and healthier lifestyle for individuals at risk;
- to enhance the security, prevent social isolation and support the multifunctional network around the individual;
- to support care providers, families and care organizations;
- to increase the efficiency and productivity of the resources in the aging societies.

This is an ongoing project with two branches: AAL+ Institutional, for institutional care; and AAL+ Home, for homecare. These are designed for continuous monitoring of health-related parameters at distance in two different scenarios, respectively: (a) *Health Institutions* (e.g. hospitals and other healthcare units, senior and assisted living residences); and (b) *Independent Living* (e.g. ambulatory and home use).

1.3 Design Principles

The project involves research and development at multiple levels, from electronics, wireless communications and embedded software (this being the main expertise of the company), to high level software targeted at healthcare professionals and end-users. Distinct features are provided in each version, so they can better respond to the intended use in each environment, typology and specific needs of the target groups. Nonetheless, AAL+ Institutional and AAL+ Home share the same base functionalities: (a) *Wireless Communications*; (b) *Continuous Monitoring*; (c) *Portability*; and (d) *Usability*.

1.3.1 Wireless Communication

In order to enhance the usability and portability of the system, the project was supported on wireless technologies, providing the desired mobility to the users. For institutional care, AAL+ Institutional provides short-to-medium range monitoring through a proprietary Radio-Frequency (RF) infrastructure setup within the facilities; residents wear wireless monitoring devices, especially designed for long-term use and adapted to their profile. For home care, AAL+ Home provides long-range monitoring over 3G cellular or wireless local area network; patients wear wireless monitoring devices that stream data in real-time through their mobile phones to a central computer.

1.3.2 Continuous Monitoring

Both versions of the system are designed to provide caregivers (doctors, nurses, orderlies, and other practitioners in general), the ability to monitor in real-time, each individual's physiological parameters throughout the day and/or receive notifications whenever anomalous conditions occur. In AAL+ Institutional, since it is intended for use within the facilities, caregivers wear special devices through which notifications are received (e.g. a subject leaving a predefined authorized perimeter generates an alarm) and summary information is shown in monitors placed at strategic locations allowing them to easily identify the individuals in need of assistance. In AAL+ Home, caregivers can observe the data collected from the patients at any given time through a web interface (e.g. activity levels, blood volume pressure). This system also allows communication with the patients to give recommendations remotely through Short Messaging Service (SMS).

1.3.3 Portability

The expected end-users for these systems belong to a highly demanding group: although continuous monitoring is an ensuring and accepted concept, these end-users are generally still very active, independent and fashionable. Together with wireless data communication, miniaturization of the devices aims to contribute for usability providing unobtrusive monitoring, enhancing the autonomy, comfort and mobility of the monitored users.

The raw materials and electronic components available nowadays, allow the creation of highly functional devices in compact and light-weighted form factors.

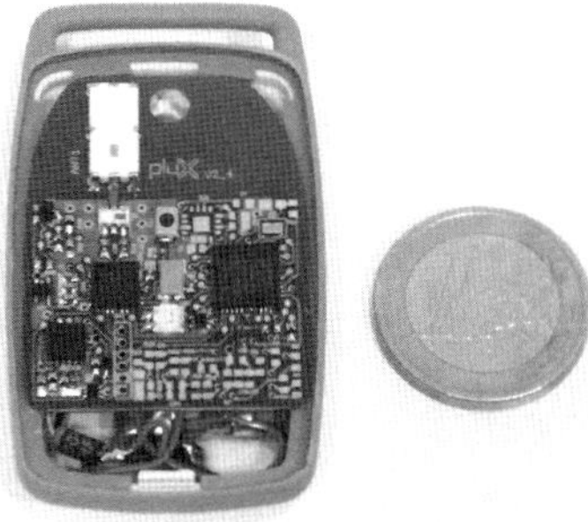

Fig. 2 AAL+ Institutional end-device size compared to a cent Euro coin (which has 16.25 mm diameter)

Figure 2 shows the relative dimensions of one AAL+ Institutional end-device prototype.

1.3.4 Integration

Caregivers are generally interested in following multiple parameters in the individuals they assist (e.g. HR and activity level), however, different functions or measurements typically require different devices. AAL+ is being developed over a modular technological basis, which enables the integration of multiple parameters into a single device. This reduces the complexity of the apparatus, increasing the applicability to other domains. From the production point of view, it allows to increase the cost-effectiveness relation since the same hardware base is used by the different devices.

2 From Research to Market

2.1 *Motivation*

Our team specialized in the development of wireless biosignal acquisition systems and sensors for healthcare and wellness applications, an example of which is the biofeedback product family for physical therapy, which is intended to provide patients with the means to expand the physical therapy training from the clinic to the home environment. In addition to this area, our R and D team works every day in new solutions for the field, being currently engaged in a series of National and EU funded projects in collaboration with other entities.

The AAL+ project arose naturally in the context of the core activities of the company, and as a result of unmet market needs. The regular activities, together with the awareness of the state-of-the-art, market analysis and the customers' needs led to this project. Two customers, one for each version of the system, were involved from the early stages, providing a clear insight about the requirements and directing the development toward the end-users real needs and acceptability criteria.

One of the customers is a Portuguese company specialized in the development of high-level software for hospital and clinical use. The services of our team were requested for the development of a portable biosignal monitoring solution, capable of providing real-time remote monitoring of activity level, Heart Rate (HR) and blood oxygenation, using a mobile phone over 3G cellular network for data transmission to a remote server located at a central hospital. This led to AAL+ Home, which base motivation was long-distance monitoring of low mobility patients suffering from chronic obstructive pulmonary disease, in order to better co-relate and adjust their oxygen consumption to their physical activity level. The goal was to optimize their oxygen prescription with less visits to the hospital.

The second client, also a Portuguese company, specialized in medical information systems, intended to develop an integrated alarm management system targeted at elderly people in Assisted Living Institutions. This led to AAL+ Institutional, its main motivation being the development of a wireless sensor network (WSN) with wearable devices for short-medium range monitoring of HR, involuntary falls and indoor location, that could automatically notify the care givers within the facility when some patient needed assistance due to some unusual condition in one of the monitored signals.

Both clients fostered interesting contacts with health institutions for test and validation of AAL+ Home and AAL+ Institutional in real world scenarios in order to assess applicability, effectiveness and usability of the systems. These contacts are allowing us to be in close contact with the end-users of the systems and better understand their needs and main difficulties right on time.

2.2 Goals

The overall goal of AAL+ is to create a modern and versatile technological basis that will be applied in the improvement of the current product line. This will allow the company to create updated versions of its products, with newer and enhanced capabilities, which are expected to contribute to the entry in new areas within the markets where the company is already operating. More specifically, AAL+ intends to give rise to a new line of products, that will enable the opportunity to address the AAL market needs, one of the currently most appealing fields within healthcare.

With a strong technological and innovation character, this is a high added value project, with expected advantages for all participants involved in its development. In general, AAL+ is resulting in reinforced notoriety within the healthcare and medical fields due to the field proven results, validated by caregivers, practitioners and end-users. We expect our customers to be able to expand their product range with the project outcomes, providing the tools for their companies to enter in novel market segments and open new commercial opportunities. Furthermore, key hardware and software technologies are being developed, whose application and potential exploitation far extend the context of the project.

Individually, for the company, AAL+ represents a big technological leap forward and an effective entrance in the area of WSN for biosignal monitoring. Additional projects that make use of the outcomes of AAL+ are already being developed to update the previously existing product lines targeted at healthcare, sports and research. As an outcome of the AAL+ development process, our engineering team is exploring in depth and expanding the state-of-the in terms of RF circuit design and protocols. This is resulting in highly energy efficient and robust systems for distributed multi-modal biosignal acquisition.

2.3 Innovation

The main innovative element of AAL+ is integration. In particular, the AAL+ Institutional equipment provides continuous monitoring of multiple patients and generation of alarms concerning indoor location, detection of falls, heart rate monitoring and panic button in the same device. On the other hand, in the case of AAL+ Home, although it may integrate, in the same system, monitoring of oximetry, cardiac and activity data, the fact that it is modular makes it extremely versatile, widening its application range.

Furthermore, our team is concerned with usability questions, both from the patient/end-user and the institution/health professional perspectives. The hardware has a small and ergonomic form factor, wireless connectivity and a pleasant appearance in order to maximize the comfort and mobility of the user. From the healthcare institutions perspective, our team is concerned also with integration of features and providing a tool with high usability. The server software keeps historic data of all patients, providing an easy way for remote follow-up and co-relation of the monitored parameters. The purpose of this feature is to help in the optimization of caregivers' time and contribute for a better quality of care.

In terms of production, multiple advances are also being motivated by the AAL+ project. Due to several optimizations in the hardware design (e.g. custom RF circuitry), the company will be able to lower the Bill of Materials (BoM) costs and plan a cost-effective production outsourcing. Other important endeavors are also arising from the project in other areas, namely in terms of Industrial Design. Together with a team of creative industrial designers and a mold engineer, custom enclosures are being created for each component of the systems, taking into account the feedback that resulted from usability tests in the partner healthcare institutions, in addition to the specific requirements of the project (e.g. inviolable bracelets for dementia patients in AAL+ Institutional). As a result, a coherent aesthetics product line that meets both form and function is being created for AAL+.

2.4 Resources

A multidisciplinary team has been involved in the project, which includes both internal and external elements to the company. Given the specificity and multi-disciplinarity of both branches of AAL+, practically all the internal team of the company has been involved, from the R&D to the Design departments. Expertise in hardware design and development, biosignal processing, telecommunications, but also in molds engineering as well as concepts of ergonomics and usability (both in the case of the hardware and the software), have been required during the development and implementation of the project. These requirements were covered entirely by the internal know-how of the company, with the ultimate goals of usability, miniaturization and portability of the devices.

In order to be successful, the project requires a close proximity with the real applicability environments and full knowledge of the patients' and caregivers' needs. Therefore, a group of external partners from the healthcare field (doctors, nurses and orderlies) was also involved in the project. These practitioners provided consultancy in the definition of requirements for AAL+ Home and AAL+ Institutional as well as in the setup and evaluation of pilot installations for functionality tests, being always in close contact with the company's internal team in order to assure the interface between the technology and its end-users.

To accomplish this task with success and to optimize the development process, the external team was expected to be well aware of the potential of using remote monitoring technologies and willing to innovate in the healthcare sector. Moreover, and since they are responsible for giving the users instructions on how to deal with the devices, they were required to have some pedagogical skills to guarantee that the users are comfortable with the devices and are capable of operating them using their full potential.

3 Continuous Institutional and Home Care Tools

3.1 AAL+ Institutional

Especially designed for assisted living facilities, the main goal of AAL+ Institutional is to provide an infrastructure for continuous short-to-medium range monitoring of location, physiological and other health-related parameters from patients, with automatic generation of alarms. This way, the early detection of critical situations is promoted, supporting institutions and caregivers in providing more efficient an effective intervention. The residents gain more independence and autonomy, and can live comfortably at the facilities feeling safe because they can call for help at any time, by knowing their biosignals are being watched, and that if any problem arises caregivers will be notified and provide assistance immediately.

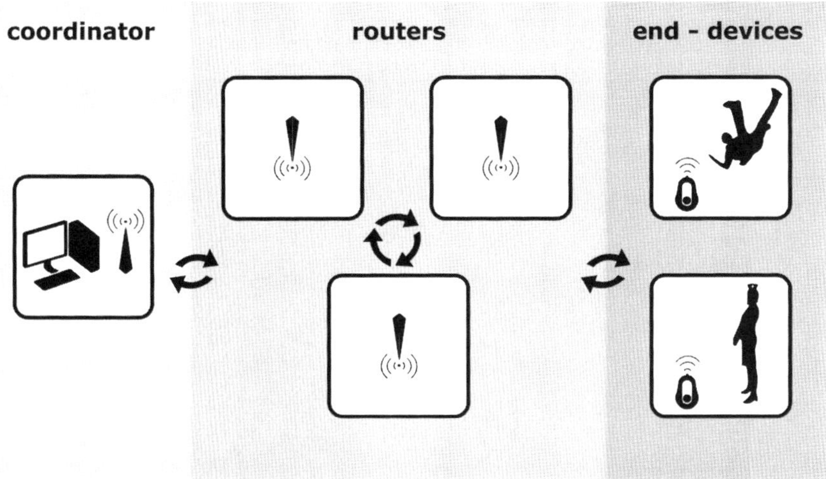

Fig. 3   AAL+ Institutional architecture

As depicted in Fig. 3, AAL+ Institutional has a WSN architecture, composed by:
(a) *Coordinator*; (b) *Routers*; and (c) *End-devices*.

3.1.1 Infrastructure

Each floor has a Linux-based central computer, to which the network coordinator
is connected, running our custom built AAL+ Network Manager server software.
This software handles all the communications going to and coming from the
network, exposing two TCP sockets that allow high-level applications to interact
with the system: (a) a *Command Socket* through which the user application can
query the network state, assign or unassign devices, manage device parameters and
query device states and measurements; and (b) an *Event Socket* through which the
use application is notified of events generated on the devices, changes in the
network state and location information.

The network routers are the fixed part of the installation, used to establish the
link between end-devices at any given location and the central computer. The
granularity that can be achieved for the location is defined by the number of
routers and their placement within the floor: fewer routers provide a rougher
insight about the location of a given end-device; more routers provide more fine
grained information. Routers have RF connectivity and are designed in such way
that they just need to be plugged to a power outlet to start operating. They forward
all the information from the end-devices to the coordinator and vice versa,
allowing caregivers to monitor heart rate, falls, location and distress calls from the
resident population in the central computer, as well as receive notifications of
impending alarms in their own personal devices.

Table 1 Technical specifications of AAL+ Institutional end-devices

	Connectivity	Resolution	Sampling Rate	Battery	Weight (g)	Size (mm)
Caregiver	868 MHz IEEE 802.15.4 Wireless	10 bit	256 Hz	Li-On; 3.7 V; 110 mAh	16	59 × 34 × 17
Wristwatch					23	57 × 43 × 17
Chest strap					43	59 × 34 × 17

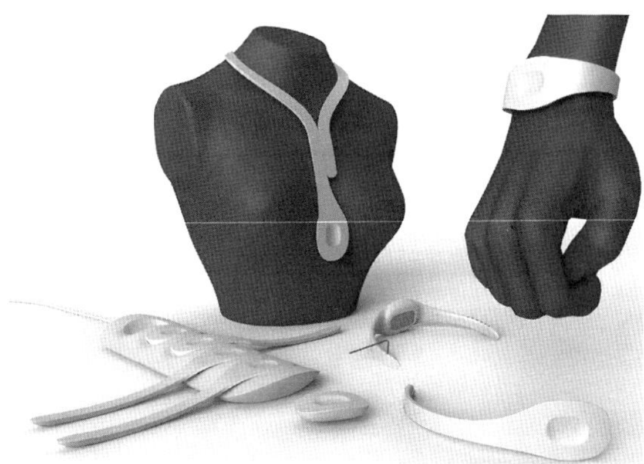

Fig. 4 Final designs of the AAL+ Institutional product family

End-devices are the wearable units that both caregivers and the monitored individuals carry with them. Although all end-devices share the same technological basis, they have different functionality and external form factors, depending on the role and profile of their end-user. Table 1 presents the main technical specifications of the end-devices.

Caregivers' devices are being designed to fit their name tags or lapel. End-user devices have additional functionalities that require contact with the person's body and are being designed to meet their usability criteria. Fig. 4 depicts the several form factor designs, which include a necklace, a wristwatch and a chest strap. The features of each device are summarized in Tables 2 and 3.

The system was engineered to meet the needs of different user profiles that can be found in AAL facilities:

- *Independent users*: highly autonomous and mobile individuals that are able to do most of their daily activities independently;
- *Dependent users*: bedridden or other individuals alike which need to be supported by others in a great majority or most of their daily activities;
- *Dementia users*: individuals with chronic or persistent disorders of the mental processes marked by memory disorders, personality changes and impaired reasoning;
- *Caregivers*: doctors, nurses, orderlies and other practitioners in general;

The end-devices, depending on their respective form factor, integrate different sensors: an Electrocardiogram (ECG) sensor, a tri-axial accelerometer and a

Table 2 AAL+ Institutional system features

End-Devices	*Features*
Chest strap	Heart rate
Necklace	Fall detection
	RF location
	Lock detection
	Manual panic button
Wristwatch	RF location
	Inviolable bracelet
	Manual panic button
Caregivers	RF Location
	Alarm acknowledgement button
Fixed nodes	
Tracking routers	Data transmission between the end-devices and the coordinator
Coordinator	Data communication between the server software and the tracking routers and end-devices

Table 3 Autonomy of each end-device type given the enabled functions

	Location call button	Location call button Fall detection	Location Call button Fall detection HR
Necklace and chest strap	2 months	11 days	3 days
Wristwatch		–	–
Caregivers			

localization module. Biosignals are automatically processed and interpreted in real-time locally, through embedded signal processing algorithms running in the devices, this includes computing the HR from the collected ECG signals and detecting acceleration patterns that can be traced back to potential fall events. Location information is provided through the WSN infrastructure itself, by using proximity information between the end-devices and the routers.

3.1.2 Alarms and Events

All the devices are fitted with a "call button" which, in the case of end-users, can be used to voluntarily issue an alarm event and request assistance, and, in the case of caregivers, is used to perform basic functions in the system (e.g. acknowledge alarms, assign or replace devices, among others). Furthermore, the necklaces and chest straps are enabled with a lock detection mechanism that triggers an alarm whenever it is opened, and wristwatches are enabled with an inviolable bracelet locking system. The AAL+ Institutional system manages two types of notifications:

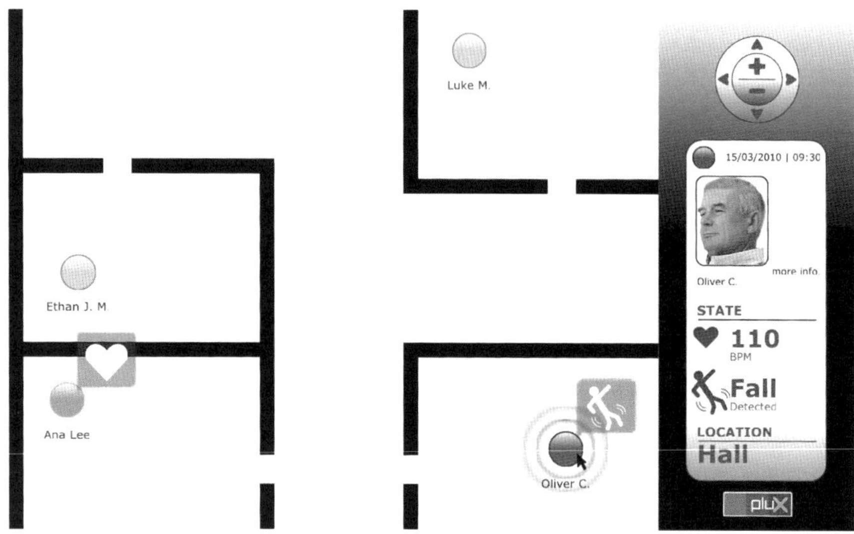

Fig. 5 Schematic representation of the user's interface of AAL+ Network Manager

- *Alarms*: which are triggered in the end-device and correspond to cases in which the HR is above or below the caregiver-defined bound, an involuntary fall is detected, or a distress call is issued through the call button;
- *Events*: which are originated both from the end-devices and the network, and correspond to responses to inquiries about location, network state, device state or HR measurements requested by the caregiver.

From the end-devices, alarms, events or explicitly requested measurements (e.g. distress call, HR values of bounds), are sent through the WSN to the central computer, allowing caregivers to be informed whenever any issue that may require their attention arises. Automatic alarms are triggered, whenever the system detects deviations of the monitored signals from the thresholds defined by caregivers as the normal condition (e.g. heart rate rising/dropping above/below a predefined threshold for each individual). Caregivers are immediately notified of alarms in their devices, where beeping signals the appearance and number of pending alarms. Patients' location and alarm typology is presented in the central station of the respective floor. Figure 5 presents a schematic representation of the central computer's AAL+ Network Manager software application.

3.1.3 Location and Communication

Location information is determined by proximity analysis, through the Received Signal Strength Indicator (RSSI). In the facilities, end-devices are, at any given time, within RF range of one, or a set of fixed nodes of the WSN. From the fixed

Table 4 Specifications of the integrated ECG sensor

Gain	1,000
Bandwidth	0.05–30 Hz
Input impedance	>100 Mohm

Table 5 Specifications of the integrated accelerometer

Number of axis	3
Measurement range	±3.6 g
X, Y, Z axis bandwidth (−3 dB)	50 Hz
Shock resistance	10,000 g

nodes within range, the end-devices determine which one has a higher RSSI value and send this information to the central station.

Given that the location of these fixed nodes within the facilities is known, the high-level software will be able to determine the perimeter in which the end-user is likely to be in. The location feature allows the system to know the approximate location of each user within the "safety perimeter" and to generate alarms when a user leaves it. If, at some moment, a given end-device is not within range of the fixed nodes, it means that it is out of the WSN bounds and an alarm is produced. Through these notifications, caregivers are able to immediately track the user and detect, for example, wandering patients leaving the facilities. This feature is particularly useful for patients with dementia.

Communication between the end-devices and the fixed nodes (coordinator and/ or routers) is done wirelessly through a 868.0 M–868.6 MHz bandwidth frequency range RF link, based on the IEEE 802.15.4 standard. Existing high-level protocols created over the IEEE 802.15.4 (e.g. ZigBee), are designed for general-purpose applications and therefore include over-engineered features for the AAL+ Institutional context. This is leading to the creation of a set of proprietary communication protocols optimized for low-power and continuous operation of the devices. Devices are powered by a 3.7 V, 110 mA h battery and Tables 3 and 4 illustrates the autonomy of the devices given the enabled functions.

3.1.4 Heart Rate and Falls

The necklace and the chest strap integrate an accelerometer and an ECG sensor. Three metallic leads fitted in the device enclosure make contact with the user's skin at the neck and at the chest levels, respectively, ensuring the proper detection of the ECG signal. The ECG is automatically processed and interpreted in real-time locally to compute the HR in the device. Table 4 summarizes the main technical specifications of the ECG sensor.

Accelerometry data is used to identify involuntary fall events. These are traced by detecting sudden changes in the magnitude of the acceleration, followed by immobilization, which triggers an alarm, ensuring that adequate assistance is rapidly provided to the user. Fall detection [7] is based on data collected in real-time

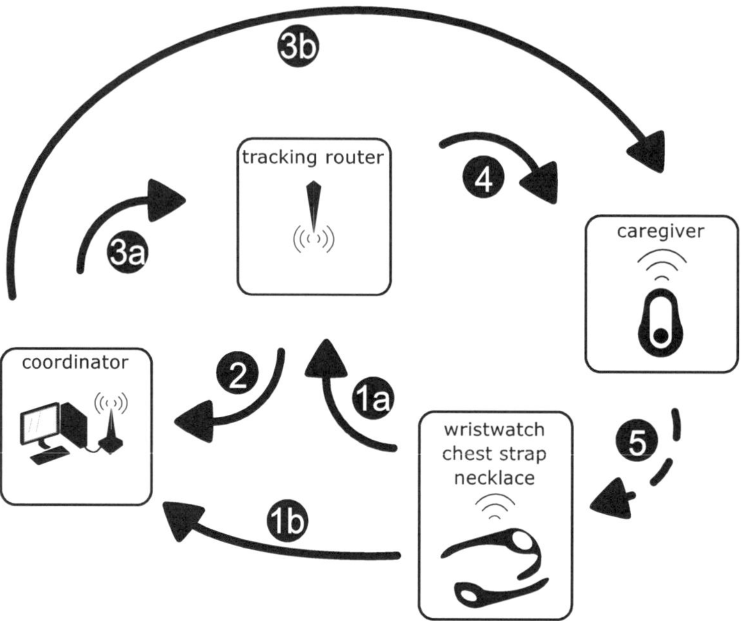

Fig. 6 Dataflow between AAL+ Institutional and center monitor elements

from a MEMS® accelerometer, integrated in the pendant part of the necklace and also in the chest strap. Table 5 summarizes the main technical specifications of the accelerometer.

In either case, information is computed in the devices from the collected raw data, through embedded signal processing algorithms and only alarms or measurements (in the case of HR) are sent through the network to the central station.

3.1.5 Data-Flow

The data flow between the devices of AAL+ Institutional is depicted in Fig. 6 and represents the overall RF interactions involved in the functioning principle of the system. When the end-devices trigger an alarm, it is forwarded to the AAL+ Network Manager Server software following one of the two pathways described below:

1. *If the device is associated with a tracking router:* The occurrence alert is first forwarded to the tracking router (Fig. 6–step 1a) and from it to the coordinator and ALL + Network Manager (Fig. 6–step 2). When the server software receives the alert, it generates an alarm and sends it to the closest caregiver device (Fig. 6–steps 3a and 4 or step 3b). This way, the caregiver is informed of the occurrence and can rapidly give the needed assistance (Fig. 6–step 5).
2. *If the device is associated directly with the coordinator:* The occurrence alert is directly sent to the coordinator and AAL+ Network Manager (Fig. 6–step 1b).

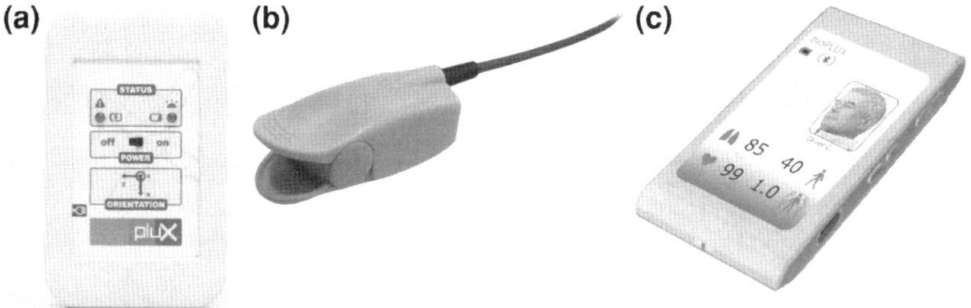

Fig. 7   AAL+ Home components

When the Network Manager server software receives the alert, it generates an alarm and sends it to the closest caregiver device (Fig. 6–steps 3a and 4 or step 3b). Finally, the caregiver acknowledges the alarm and helps the user (Fig. 6–step 5).

3.2 AAL+ Home

Especially designed for home care and independent living, the main goal of AAL+ Home is to provide an infrastructure for continuous long range biosignal monitoring in near real-time. This version of the AAL+ project aims the development of a wearable system, that can be used by patients at their homes and throughout their day-to-day activities, continuously monitoring parameters such as physical activity level, HR or blood oxygenation level. The system is targeted mainly at senior users who still maintain their full mental capabilities and independence, but for some reason need ambulatory, long-range monitoring of the referred parameters. However, the system applicability is broader; the team believes that AAL+ Home will contribute for promoting a healthier lifestyle for people in general and also help in maintaining wellness, autonomy and functional capability of people in other risk groups, such as chronic respiratory or obese patients. This is a modular telehealth system conceived with both caregivers and patients in mind.

3.2.1 Infrastructure

Depending on the monitoring needs of each subject, one or more independent wireless sensor nodes are worn by the end-users for biosignal acquisition (e.g. activity monitor, pulse oximeter); subjects also carry a cellular phone with them that operates as a mobile gateway, interfacing the wireless sensor nodes with the remote monitoring station. The mobile gateway also provides local on-screen visualization of the main indicators (e.g. HR, oxygen saturation level), which allows the end-user to use it as a mobile phone based self-management tool. Fig. 7 illustrates the wireless sensor nodes and mobile gateway.

a. Wireless Tri-axial Accelerometer.
b. Wireless Pulse Oximeter.
c. Mobile Gateway.

A software running in the mobile gateway collects the data in real-time from the wireless sensor nodes via Bluetooth$^{®}$ RF connection, streaming it to the remote monitoring station through TCP/IP socket connection over cellular 3G or 802.11 WiFi network. An intrinsic problem in mobile communication is the fact that mobile devices can be frequently out of network coverage (e.g. a person traveling in a subway or in an elevator); in general there are no guarantees regarding the network coverage. For this purpose, the software on the mobile gateway is enabled with data buffering and re-transmission capabilities; also, basic signal processing and packet encoding tasks are performed in order to optimize the channel payload for more efficient communications management.

The remote monitoring station is an Internet-enabled computer installed at the healthcare institution, running a MySQL relational database management system and our own server-side software application, in charge of managing the socket connections and all incoming data from each mobile gateway. Their mobile gateway phone number identifies end-users and the data received on the remote monitoring station is stored in the database and associated to the corresponding patient record. Caregivers can visualize in near real-time the data from each end-user stored on the database through a web interface, which also allows them to configure the system (e.g. define the regular bounds for the measurements taken by each wireless sensor node) and send communicate with the end-users.

3.2.2 Alarms and Messaging

AAL+ Home intends to bridge the communication gap between the clinician and the end-user when they are away from the healthcare institution, while providing an efficient method for the early detection or prevention of potentially anomalous situations. Furthermore, notifications are sent to the remote monitoring station, which are issued when one of the following cases is detected on any of the devices worn by the end-user: (a) *lost connection*; (b) *low battery*; or (c) *incorrect sensor placement*.

Through the web interface, clinicians receive alarms and notifications whenever the measurements coming from the wireless sensor nodes come out of the previously specified bounds, or whenever a relevant state change occurs either in the mobile gateway or in the wireless sensor nodes. Moreover, clinicians can send SMSs to the end-users giving them advice concerning the optimization of the monitored parameters. End-users on the other hand, may voluntarily generate alarm messages by pressing a pre-defined key on the mobile gateway, in order to remotely request for assistance from the caregivers.

Table 6 Specifications of activity level node BP motion

Connectivity	Class II bluetooth® connectivity; 10 m range
Resolution	12 bit
Sampling rate	1,000 Hz
Measurement range	3 axis
Measurement range	±3 G
Weight	74 g
Dimensions	84 × 53 × 18 mm
Battery	Li-On; 7.4 V; 800 mAh

Table 7 Activity levels classification according to the MET values

MET value	Intensity of the activity
<= 3	Light
3 > MET > 6	Moderate
MET > 6	Vigorous

Table 8 Technical specifications of the pulse oximeter

IR wavelength	870 nm
RED wavelength	635 nm
Bandwidth $(-3\ dB)$	0.5–6 Hz

3.2.3 Activity Level and Blood Oxygen Saturation

Although the system can be expanded to include other variables, in its current configuration activity levels and blood oxygen saturation are measured. Activity levels are monitored by a portable and highly miniaturized wireless tri-axial accelerometer, designed for waist placement, and continuously monitoring the end-user throughout day. The device is shown in Fig. 7a and its technical specifications are listed in Table 6.

Acceleration magnitude is directly co-related with the physical activity intensity level, and can be expressed in "Counts" and "MET" units. Counts are the base physical activity measurement unit provided by the system and converted in METs ("Metabolic Equivalent of Task"), which is a standard unit to characterize energy expenditure in physical activities. [8–10] The conversion of "Counts" to "MET" is performed on the AAL+ Home mobile gateway, through a non-linear signal processing algorithm with two regression equations relating "Counts"; "MET" values are determined based on the method by Crouter et. al. [11] Table 7 shows the physical activity level as classified according to the respective MET value [8].

Blood oxygen saturation (SpO2) and heart rate (HR) are monitored by a pulse oximeter. For development, our team is using a third-party, wrist worn device with a finger clip sensor and Bluetooth connectivity, that transmits the data in real-time to the mobile phone. Currently there is a Bluetooth finger clip sensor under development, depicted in Fig. 7b, which is based on our current sensor,

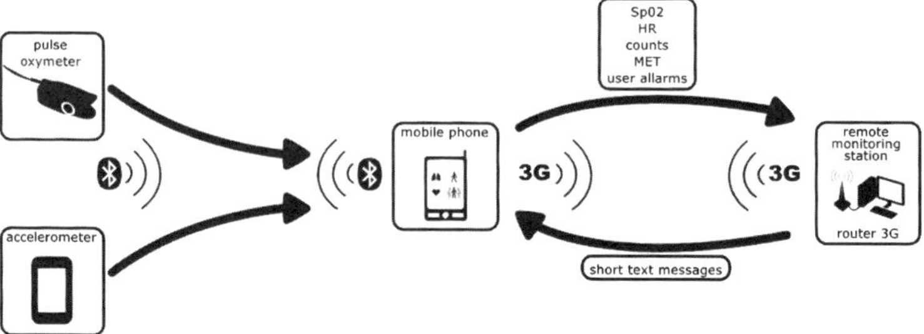

Fig. 8 Data-flow between AAL+ Home components

that will be used for this purpose. Table 8 presents the technical specifications of this sensor.

3.2.4 Data-Flow

The relation between the wireless sensor nodes, mobile gateway and the remote monitoring station is represented in Fig. 8. Wireless sensor nodes measure the raw data at different sampling rates (1,000 Hz for the accelerometer; and 200 Hz for the pulse oximeter) and send it in real-time via Bluetooth to the mobile gateway, where they are buffered and processed. Counts, METs, SpO2 and HR data are continuously shown on-screen at the mobile gateway and, from there, transmitted in real-time over 3G cellular or WiFi network to the remote monitoring station, where caregivers can observe it through the web interface, providing a means to quickly detect problems and take the necessary actions. Alarms and notification generated in the mobile gateway and SMSs sent to it by caregivers are also sent through the same channel.

Each user has its own mobile gateway and wireless sensor nodes set that are fully configured remotely. Data synchronization is assured through the remote monitoring station, which periodically sends the central server time to the mobile gateway, allowing all the data collected from the different end-users to be on the same time base. Also, a handshaking protocol was developed for transactional management of the transmitted data; together with the buffering capabilities of the mobile gateway, this avoids data loss due to network coverage or communication problems. Two conditions may be found in which the remote monitoring station signals the mobile gateway:

1. *Successful transmission*: where a message is sent to clear the buffered data;
2. *Erroneous transmission*: where a message is sent requesting retransmission and with the indication of the point-of-failure.

When a new connection is established, the remote monitoring station reads the configuration data for that end-user from the database (wireless sensor nodes MAC addresses, required measurements and communication period) and remotely configures the mobile gateway accordingly.

3.3 Advantages

AAL+ is bringing important benefits for the reality of healthcare institutions, caregivers and end-users. These generally translate into higher efficiency, faster intervention in anomalous situations, more effective delivery of care, and subsequent cost reduction throughout the process. The system has advantages for all agents.

For institutions, the system brings: (a) greater management control; (b) more effective resource planning; (c) higher efficiency due to intervention models; (d) increased customer satisfaction; and (e) notoriety due to technological lead. For example, in the AAL+ Institutional pilot, the system provides the facility with indicators which otherwise would not be readily available, as the caregivers response time to alarms. This allows them to increase to quality of labor, by identifying critical parts of the processes and improving them.

For caregivers, the system brings: (a) convenience of monitoring end-users at distance; (b) faster identification of anomalous situations through the automated alarms and notifications; (c) improved communication with their counterparts through the clinical records; and (d) possibility of monitoring multiple end-users in parallel. For example, prior to the installation of the AAL+ Institutional pilot caregivers would regularly go to each individual to take HR measurements; through the system they were able to take the same measurements remotely and automatically, reducing the number of visits to end-users and allowing them to manage the time more efficiently.

For patients, the system brings: (a) improved quality of life; (b) higher sense of security due to continuous monitoring and automated alarm generation; (c) receive faster assistance in case of anomalous situations; (d) conveniently request assistance in any circumstance. For example, in the case of AAL+ Home, the system is expected to reduce the number of control visits that patients make to the hospital as well as the number of admissions due to the fact that they are more closely controlled.

4 User-Centric Development

4.1 Field Tests

Two pilot installations, one for each version, have already been setup for functional tests in a real environment. During its development, AAL+ Institutional was deployed in two different stages at an Assisted Living Residence for the elderly. An early prototype was tested on a total of three residents accompanied by one caregiver for a period of 6 months. As a result of these initial tests, valuable information was collected, namely at usability and network infrastructure configuration levels. Regarding usability, tests revealed the need to improve on the fabrics and method for attaching the devices to the users body. In terms of network infrastructure, this early version of the system relied on 802.15.4 RF modules with a ZigBee protocol compliant stack, operating in the 2.4 GHz frequency. These revealed to perform poorly due to the proliferation of and overcrowded spectrum due the proliferation of 802.11 WiFi networks operating in the same frequency in different channels.

Taking into account the test results, an improved version of the system was created using custom designed RF modules operating in the 868 MHz frequency and with a proprietary communication protocol developed at IEEE 802.15.4 MAC layer. A pre-production version of this system was later successfully tested on a wider group of 13 residents accompanied by five caregivers for a period of 4 months. The network infrastructure was composed of a central computer, ten tracking routers and one coordinator ensured the network coverage of four wings of the building and existing common areas. Final results have shown the acceptance and usability of the improved system design and adopted solutions for long term usage by the elderly population. The new network infrastructure proved to overcome the initially identified issues.

AAL+ Home has been fully deployed at a major Portuguese hospital allowing the doctors to remotely monitor 30 patients at any given time. The selected test group is composed by patients with severe respiratory insufficiency under long-term oxygen therapy, which required periodic follow-up visits to the hospital unit in a weekly basis. For these patients travels are extremely demanding and in between appointments their contact with the doctors was extremely limited. AAL+ Home pilot started operating in December 2009 and it is currently still in use with successful results due to valences that it introduced in the existing reality.

The fact that doctors have real-time access to accurate diagnosis data and alarms, together with a direct communication channel, allows them to instantly send instructions and recommendations to the patients' mobile phones (e.g. adjust the debit of the oxygen bottle). Patients and their families have gained in quality of life. Since they are continuously monitored, fewer visits to the hospital are required and as the patient's therapy is more closely accompanied by doctors in between visits to the hospital, the frequency in admissions due to anomalous situations has also decreased.

4.2 Training

Both versions of the AAL+ system require that end-users and caregivers receive basic usage instructions. For the pilot installations, support documentation was prepared (e.g. user manual) and an initial training was delivered to caregivers. This training was performed on-site and focused on essential aspects related to each system, covering issues that ranged from the features available in each device, to alarm management, device assignment and replacement procedures, cleansing and charging. In either case caregivers or other designated practitioners were in charge of instructing the end-users and guiding them through the usage process.

In the case of AAL+ Home, other agents besides caregivers and end-users may become involved in the operation of the system, since many times, patients at home can have relatives and/or other individuals assisting them in their daily routines. For this system a quick guide was prepared, summarizing in a few simple and straightforward steps, the most elementary information regarding the regular usage of the devices. This includes connecting, disconnecting and charging the wireless sensor nodes and mobile gateway, interpreting the on-screen data and SMS visualization.

With other market opportunities in mind, technical documentation was also produced for partners that want to integrate AAL+ in their own solutions. For them, the company created a set of API reference guides, protocol description and diagrams that easily assist third-party companies through the core aspects of the system in a developer point of view.

4.3 Usability

The users' acceptability tests performed for AAL+ Home and AAL+ Institutional show that usability is one a key issues in projects in this area: the user needs to be capable of understand all features of the equipments so that the full potentialities of the remote monitoring may be used.

End-users are here seen from two different perspectives: (a) the patients; (b) the caregivers and their satisfaction is one of the main goals of the project.

Patients are satisfied if they feel comfortable and safe wearing the continuous monitoring equipments and if their independence and autonomy are not compromised with the process.

On the other hand, the caregivers aim to have tools that enable them to optimize their time and provide better and faster assistance to the patients.

With this in mind, the team has been concerned in creating non-intrusive and practical hardware, fulfilling users' requirements of miniaturization, ergonomic design and water resistance. In order to reach these goals molding industry is also being involved in the project so that the final appearance of the devices is pleasant and comfortable to wear, enhancing this way patients' satisfaction.

Moreover, the team is engaged in the creation of intuitive and user-friendly software applications for both branches of the project so that interpretation of the presented data is straightforward, this way further enhancing the caregivers' performance.

4.4 The User in the Loop

Due to its nature and objective, the project is being developed under a user-centric approach, where prototypes are closely validated in the field and undergo an

Fig. 9 AAL+ Institutional
prototype devices

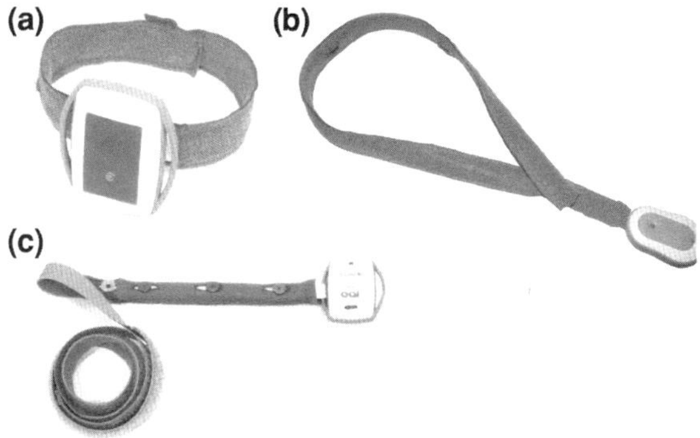

extensive set of usability tests. Each version of the system has a different impact in
the end-users routines and distinct levels of intrusiveness.

AAL+ Home is a discrete system that involves moderate contact with the
person's body. When only the activity levels are measured the end-users are just
required to wear a mobile phone and the miniaturized wireless accelerometer. Both
of these devices have neoprene sleeves and are fitted to a belt that the person
places around the waist making it a practical system for regular use. The pulse
oximeter requires a finger clip sensor to be placed on the index or middle finger
and has a wrist watch alike form factor. During the field tests performed with the
system, users generally expressed positive reactions to the system in terms of
portability and usability. However, the pulse oximeter apparatus and size were
pointed out as possible improvement points; for this reason, a new and highly
integrated sensor is currently under development that will allow provide the same
functionality in a more compact formfactor.

For AAL+ Institutional devices were designed taking into account the specificity of each end-user profile and the intended use. Devices were intended for
continuous use in contact with the persons' body, which forced us to create
watertight enclosures that end-users can wear even while they are showering, as
well as washable materials and surfaces. Caregiver devices were designed to fit the
uniforms and apparel normally used by the professionals. Wrist watches were
fitted with an inviolable bracelet in order to prevent their target users (dementia
patients) from removing the devices. Both of these devices were well received
during the pilot tests.

The necklace and chest strap versions, however, have gone through multiple
refinement steps; these are devices whose measured parameters and intended use
requires firm contact with the body for long periods of time. Early prototypes are
depicted in Fig. 9. In their initial stage, field tests revealed that necklaces were
poorly received by women as they interfered aesthetically with elements such as
jewellery and clothing necklines. Chest straps, on the other hand, presented fas-
tening problems and after a few hours of use would slip down the subject's upper
body.

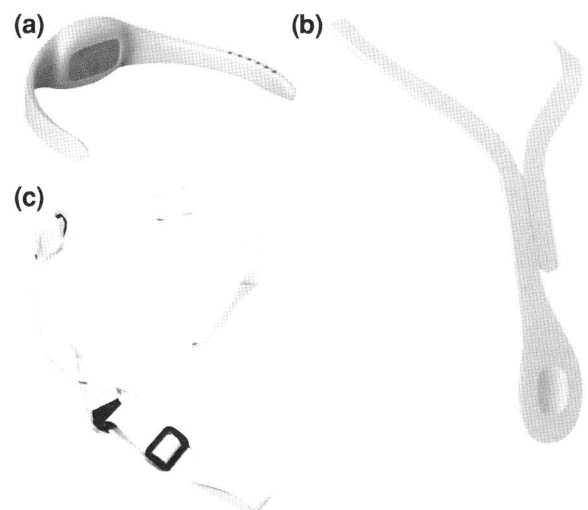

Fig. 10 AAL+ Institutional final devices

a. Wristwatch.
b. Necklace.
c. Chest Strap.

Results from these tests were used to develop improved and more robust solutions. Together with textile engineers, special sleeves were developed for the devices, solving the identified issues. The necklaces are slipped into textile sleeves that give them the look-and-feel of another clothing accessory and the chest straps have a textile sleeve with a shoulder loop that prevents them from slipping of place. Figure 10 depicts the final version.

a. Wristwatch.
b. Necklace.
c. Chest Strap.

5 Socioeconomic Factors

5.1 Regional Context

Portugal has a highly critical and well aware population in terms of international trends, being known for early technological adoption as demonstrated, among others, by indicators as the high penetration rate of mobile phones [12], and the recent Magalhães (Magellan) initiative for widespread ICT access in schools [13]. Therefore, the valuable inputs and insight provided by this market allow the outcomes of the project to compete at a global scale in its late development and final version stages, while lowering the benchmarking and validation costs in the early specification and development stages.

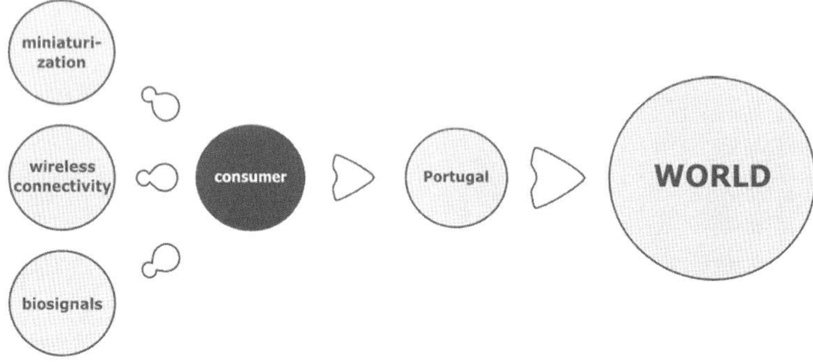

Fig. 11 Product development policy

The company has a R&D policy of using Portugal as the initial platform for project development and experimentation. Figure 11 depicts this process. Given its proximity to the Portuguese market and the expertise found in multiple technical and medical fields, it is possible to benchmark, test and validate the developed products with well-recognized experts at a global level. Through this direct contact with elements from both academia and *praxis*, the team is able to maximize the convergence of AAL+ specifications and features to the effective overall market needs and demands.

5.2 Economic Impact

AAL+ is the result of the company's internal R&D activities, with a multidisciplinary team of experts allocated to the project gathering know-how from engineering, management and quality. Both for AAL+ Institutional and AAL+ Home, the services contracted by our customers for initial proof-of-concept and pilot facilities installation have allowed us not only to financially leverage the project development during its early stages, but also gave us the opportunity to validate intermediate results in close collaboration with end-users and healthcare professionals in the field.

Furthermore, the project was partially supported by funding from qualification and innovation projects submitted to the National Strategic Reference Framework (NSRF–QREN) agenda. Through an approved project in the area of Certification, the company was able to initiate the implementation of a Quality Management System (QMS), that was extended to the documentation, versioning and control of the AAL+ project. Moreover, this NSRF project is also enabling the preparation of Technical Files and the implementation of the necessary procedures for Production Quality Management that must be submitted to the Notified Body for CE marking of the outcomes of AAL+ as medical devices.

Activities from other approved NSRF projects have also introduced important contributions in the development of AAL+. Their outcomes have contributed to the project not only in terms of R&D, but also in areas such as marketing, promotion and results dissemination in scientific forums [14].

5.3 Legal and Regulatory Aspects

As a medical devices manufacturer, the company must follow specific legislation issued and highly regulated by health authorities so that the resulting products may be placed on the market. Although other markets are also in study, the outcomes of the project will be initially explored within the European market. Within the European Community (EC), in order for a product to be placed in the market it must comply with the applicable regulations and directives. Depending on the nature of the product, different directives must be chosen. Given the intended function of the AAL+ products, they fall in the definition of a medical device. Therefore, in order to be placed on the market they must comply with all the Essential Requirements of the European Medical Directive (Directive 2007/47/ EC), [15, 16] pass a specific conformity assessment procedure and have the CE Mark affixed on it.

The development of AAL+ is following the quality, safety and performance principles adopted by the company, as defined by the essential requirements of the Medical Directive to which the products resultant from the project must comply when used for the intended purposes. Special design considerations are being followed by the team, which include:

- General requirements for safe design.
- Minimization of risks from contamination.
- Compatibility of materials with which the devices is likely to be in contact.
- Minimization of hazards of infection and microbial contamination.
- Provision of sufficient accuracy.
- Protection against radiation and electrical shock.
- Adequate product labeling and user instructions.

A technical file that contains information demonstrate that the devices and related accessories comply with the MDD according to the conformity procedure chosen is being created for both AAL+ Institutional and AAL+ Home products in parallel with the R and D process. This document includes detailed description of the devices and manufacturing procedure, risk analysis, test and validation reports, list of applied standards and QMS support documentation.

Moreover, the company is undergoing through the preparation for the implementation of its QMS, according to the International Standard Organization (ISO), whose procedures and regulatory recommendations are assisting the project at multiple levels: ISO 9001:2008 [17] standard is guiding the establishment of methods for enhanced continuous improvement processes and the assurance of conformity to the customer and applicable regulations; ISO 13485:2003 [18] is contributing for the design of procedures related to the production of medical devices and related services; and ISO 14971:2007 [19] is providing the tools for risk and hazard management throughout the life of AAL+ products.

5.4 Dissemination Strategy

AAL+ is being actively promoted; as an R&D project, intermediate results are frequently published in national and international scientific forums. Also, the company regularly participates in trade fairs and events where the working prototypes are demoed and explained to interested visitors. Furthermore, direct contact with institutions in the field and promotion within our partners network are also mechanisms that the company uses to disseminate the outcomes and prospects of the project.

6 Conclusion

In an ageing and increasingly more demanding society with growing life expectancy, the development of tools that enhance the management of healthcare and clinical monitoring are in valuable in order to optimize the performance of assistance given to patients. According to the Eurostat [3] in 2060 there will be only two people of working age for every person aged over 65 years old, contrasting to 2008, when the ratio was of 4:1. As a consequence one should expect to see a decrease in the availability of medical practitioners, while the affluence to hospitals will increase, also increasing the waiting times and pressure in hospitals and other clinical facilities. The implementation of remote monitoring solutions will, therefore, not only enhance the quality of life for patients and end-users as they are more closely controlled, but also enhance the quality of care provided by caregivers and institutions as more rigorous data and automated alarm tools become available for real-time assessment of the end-user condition.

The AAL+ project aims to contribute for these enhancements in peoples' lives, providing tools for convenient monitoring of health related parameters at distance in Institutional and at Home scenarios. For this purpose, the project is being developed under two branches: (a) AAL+ Institutional for healthcare institutions; and (b) AAL+ Home for independent living. A multidisciplinary development team has been involved in this project, ranging from hardware engineers and researchers, to designers and clinical practitioners, in order to take into account not only technical specifications and performance, but also usability and user acceptability questions, which in the area of AAL applications are of great importance in order to the make project succeeded.

After the initial stages of development and deployment in real world pilot installations, both versions of the system are currently in a late prototype stage. Experimental results from the functional and usability tests reveal that there are multiple advantages brought by the introduction of these technologies, which extend to institutions, caregivers and end-users and translate into faster assistance to users, higher efficiency of the services and novel intervention models.

Acknowledgments This work was partially supported by the National Strategic Reference Framework (NSRF–QREN) programme under contracts no. 3,494, 4,329 and 7,900 (respectively: i2Life, Internationalization and Living Usability Lab for Next Generation Networks) and by Fundação Portuguesa para a Ciência e Tecnologia (FCT) under grant SFRH/BD/65248/2009, whose support the authors gratefully acknowledge.

References

1. U.S. Census Bureau. 2008 National population projections. [Online]. 2008. Available from: http://www.census.gov/population/www/projections/2008projections.html.
2. Organization for economic co-operation and development (OECD). OECD Factbook 2009: economic, environmental and social statistics. Paris: OECD Publishing; 2009.
3. Konstantinos G. Ageing characterises the demographic perspectives of the European societies. Eurostat Statistics in Focus 2008; 72/2008.
4. Yogesan K, Brett P, Gibbons MC, editors. Handbook of digital homecare. Berlin: Springer; 2007.
5. Aziz D, Lo B, Pansiot J, Atallah L, Yang G, Darzy A. From computers to ubiquitous computing by 2010: health care. Phil Trans R Soc A. 2008;366(1881):3805–3811.
6. Ambient assisted living (AAL). [Online]. Available from: http://www.aal-europe.eu/about-aal.
7. Silva H, Silva F, Gamboa H, Viegas V. Automatic fall detection and alert system - a compact GPS/GSM enabled unit based on accelerometry. Proc. of BIODEVICES 2008 Jan 2.
8. Wikipedia–the free encyclopedia. Metabolic equivalent [Online] 2010. Available from: http://en.wikipedia.org/wiki/Metabolic_equivalent.
9. Ainsworth BE, Haskell WL, Leon AS, Jacobs DR Jr, Montoye HJ, Sallis JF, Paffenbarger RS Jr. Compendium of physical activities: classification of energy costs of human physical activities. Med Sci Sports Exerc. 1993;25:71–80.
10. Ainsworth BE, Haskell WL, Whitt MC, Irwin ML, Swartz AM, Strath SJ, O'Brien WL, Bassett DR Jr, Schmitz KH, Emplaincourt PO, Jacobs DR Jr, Leon AS. Compendium of physical activities: an update of activity codes and MET intensities. Med Sci Sports Exerc. 2000;32(Suppl):S498–516.
11. Crouter SE, Clowers KG, Bassett DR Jr. A novel method for using accelerometer data to predict energy expenditure. J Appl Pysiol. 2006;100:1324–31.
12. Nationmaster. Mobile phones by country [Online]. 2003. Available from: http://www.nationmaster.com/graph/med_mob_pho-media-mobile-phones.
13. Intel Press Release. Intuitive convertible design for the intel-powered classmate PC enhances collaborative learning [Online]. 2009 Jan 9. Available from: http://www.intel.com/pressroom/archive/releases/2009/20090109comp.htm.
14. Gamboa H, Silva F, Silva H. Patient tracking system. Proceedings of pervasive health conference 2010; 2010 Mar 22–5, Munich.
15. Directive 2007/47/EC of the European parliament and of the council of 5 Sept 2007.
16. http://eurlex.europa.eu/LexUriServ/LexUriServ.do?uri=OJ:L:2007:247:0021:0055:en:PDF.

17. ISO 9001:2008 Quality man. System requirements, http://www.iso.org/iso/iso_9001_2008.
18. ISO 13485:2003 Medical device - quality management standard, http://www.iso.org/iso/catalogue_detail?csnumber=36786.
19. ISO 14971:2007 Medical devices – application of risk management to medical devices, http://www.iso.org/iso/catalogue_detail.htm?csnumber=38193.

Home Medication Management by Videophone: Translation from Pilot Project to Integrated Service

Victoria A. Wade, Angela Littleford and Debbie Kralik

Abstract The implementation of a telehomecare medication management service, by a community health and care organisation, is described from pilot project to ongoing service. Nurses undertake virtual visits using videophones to guide and monitor medication administration for home-based clients with cognitive impairment, or for those receiving directly observed therapy for tuberculosis. Changes in nursing roles, the development of new clinical protocols and procedures, and a new method of providing flexible, high bandwidth connectivity to the home were developed. Clients reported the telehealth service to be convenient, reassuring, and less intrusive than face-to-face contact, and found the videophones easy to operate. The nursing service found the telehealth service was safe, reliable, cost-effective, and that clients improved their health status. The translation to service integration was accomplished by dedicated resourcing, staff education, addressing staff concerns, the development of a telehealth unit, and a clinical–technical partnership. The critical organizational success factors were the engagement of clinicians, clear development of new professional roles, a continuing change management strategy, and leadership.

Keywords Telehomecare · Videophone · Medication management · Community nursing

V. A. Wade (✉)
Discipline of Public Health, The University of Adelaide, Adelaide, SA, Australia
e-mail: victoria.wade@adelaide.edu.au

A. Littleford · D. Kralik
The Royal District Nursing Service of South Australia, Adelaide, SA, Australia

Commun Med Care Compunetics (2011) 3: 143–165
DOI: 10.1007/8754_2011_26
© Springer-Verlag Berlin Heidelberg 2011
Published Online: 14 May 2011

1 Description of the Project

This project developed and implemented a service to supervise home medication administration by nurses using videophones. The hosting organization, the Royal District Nursing Service of South Australia Inc (RDNS SA) is the major community nursing and care service in metropolitan Adelaide, a city of about 1.3 million people. RDNS SA provides health services in people's homes, where nurses visit clients and provide the care required, or under supervision of a registered nurse, care workers follow prescribed care plans which are carefully monitored. In addition to home-based services RDNS SA has clinics in a variety of metropolitan locations, some of which are co-located with other services such as a pharmacy chain. RDNS SA has approximately 21,000 active clients with 1,600 admissions and discharges every month, and medication supervision is frequently provided by the home visiting service.

1.1 History of the Project

The telehealth project began in 2007, when RDNS SA initiated a 6 month trial of videophone technology to deliver medication management in a community setting. The trial was partly funded by a small grant from the South Australian Department of Health, which covered the equipment and connectivity costs, and was also internally supported by RDNS SA, by allocating staff time for implementation. Nine clients who needed medication supervision, but did not require hands-on nursing services, had Digital Services Lines (DSL, also known as "broadband") and home videophones installed, and their drive-around visits were replaced by virtual visits. The nurses conducting the virtual visits were based within the existing RDNS SA call centre, which operates 24 hours a day, 7 days a week, and this centre also had two videophones installed for the project. As client numbers were small, these additional virtual visits were added to the nurses' usual duties. The trial was successfully completed and evaluated, showing that the technology was reliable, suitable, safe, equitable, cost-effective, accepted by clients, and provided benefits to clients, their families and healthcare professionals [1]. Throughout 2008 virtual visits were maintained as a service option for this small group of clients, whilst business and strategic planning for telehealth took place, and in 2009 a new telehealth unit was formed within the call centre, with positions created for additional nursing staff. By the end of March 2010 there were 73 clients receiving the service.

1.2 Clients of the Project

Two types of clients are entered into this service:

1. People with cognitive impairment, who live alone and need assistance to take their medication correctly and safely. The majority of people in this group have age-related dementia with multiple other chronic conditions, and a minority have alcohol related brain damage, post-head injury memory impairment, and/ or mental health issues.
2. People who are receiving Directly Observed Therapy (DOT) for tuberculosis. This group are referred by the Chest Clinic run by the South Australian Department of Health, and are those clients with tuberculosis for whom there are some concerns about the likelihood of adherence to the full course of treatment.

1.3 Operations of the Project

Clients with cognitive impairment receive a gradual introduction to the telehealth service; initially they have a daily in-home visit with a nurse who guides and instructs them in the use of the videophone. As the client becomes more proficient the nurse gradually reduces his/her support until the client is using the equipment and taking the medications with the assistance of the nurse at the other end of the videophone. All these clients need to have their medication in a sealed administration aid; the specific type utilized in this service is the Webster pack. If the client is not currently using an administration aid this is commenced before introducing the videophone, and the field nurse conducts 'prompt' visits for a minimum of 2 weeks to educate the client in the use of the pack and to ensure familiarity and dexterity. After the videophone is installed, nurses still do one in-home visit per week for these clients, to check that the Webster pack contents correlate with the medication authority provided by the prescribing doctor, and that this authority is up to date. In addition to monitoring the clients' administration of their medication, nurses also check the clients' disposition, and as they are in frequent contact, are readily able to detect early signs of illness or functional deterioration. In general, the virtual visits are initiated from the call centre, although a minority of clients will call in first. This service is intended for long-term clients, and whilst length of requirement cannot be predicted, some clients have now received the service for over 2 years.

For clients receiving DOT, only one home visit is needed, to deliver and install the videophone, and from then on all their visits are virtual. This group does not require their medications in an administration aid, and about half of these clients initiate the video calls themselves. They are able to call in any time between 5 am and 11 pm. The usual length of service is between 6 and 12 months, which is the duration of the anti-tubercular treatment.

All episodes of medication ingestion are observed by the service. The most frequently prescribed medication regimen was found to be twice daily, for 44% of clients, followed by daily medication (35%), three times a day (15%), and four times a day (5%).

2 Development of the Project

The broad argument for developing this project is that telehealth is an increasingly well researched method of providing home healthcare [2] with studies finding that health outcomes can be improved in hypertension, diabetes, asthma and heart failure [3–6]. Whilst the majority of these programs are for specific chronic diseases, it was felt that there was good potential to adapt the telehealth model to medication management of diverse conditions, and implement a safe alternative for clients requiring assistance with medication administration.

2.1 The Problem of Medication Adherence

Finding new ways to improve medication adherence is important because non-adherence is a substantial problem in healthcare, resulting in increased deaths, worsening of disease, and increases in health care costs [7]. In the United States, medication errors in older people were estimated to cost $US 177 billion per year, and if they were counted as a disease, would be the fifth leading cause of death for Americans older than 65 [8].

For the whole of population, adherence rates vary from quite low to around 80%. In a very large sample of over 600,000 people in the US, the adherence rates for chronic conditions were about 80% for anti-hypertensives, and 77% for oral diabetes medications [9]. The 45,678 participants in the European Social Survey also self-reported approximately 80% adherence [10], however caution should be applied in the interpretation of these results as self reported data over-estimates adherence [7]. Average rates of adherence in community-based clinical trials varied from 43 to 78% for patients receiving treatment for chronic conditions and is also likely to over-estimate adherence, due to the selection and additional monitoring patients receive in a trial [7]. In general, adherence is worse for patients with chronic conditions [11].

Hospital admissions are one of the costly consequences of medication problems: between 33 and 69% of all medication related admissions to hospital in the US are due to poor medication adherence, with an estimated cost of $100 billion a year [7]. Approximately 140,000 hospital admissions a year in Australia are due to medication problems, which is under 5% of total admissions, but this number rises to 30% of admissions in people aged over 75 years. It is notable that 69% of these admissions were classified as preventable [12]. Frail older people who need assistance with medication management but do not receive it are at higher risk of hospitalization [13].

Medication management is a substantial proportion of the work of community nursing and home care services [14], and in elderly populations receiving these services studies have found non-adherence rates ranging from 64% for clients of a home healthcare agency [15], 62% for community-dwelling disabled older persons [13], to 12.5% (self-reported) in people over 65 receiving health or social services [16]. In general, older people living at home have more medication related misadventure than those in nursing homes [17], and the greatest predictors of non-adherence are problem drinking, lack of medical review, and cognitive impairment [16].

Much of the literature on implementing solutions in this area is from the USA, because government funding of home care agencies serving people aged 65 and over requires that their clients are assessed for ability to manage medications [8], and that the agencies' medication management outcomes are reported [14]. This, plus recognition of the consequences of non-adherence has led to quality improvement initiatives in the area, however, telehealth does not appear to have reached the mainstream, and is not mentioned, for example, in the recent National Framework for Geriatric Home Care Excellence [8].

Despite the substantial nature and costly effects of non-adherence, research to date has not found solutions that effectively deal with the problem. Analysis of reviews of adherence to medical treatment indicate that many complex and time-consuming interventions have only modest effects [13]. A Cochrane review of 93 studies on improving medication adherence for medical problems, which only included studies measuring patient health outcomes [18], reported that 44% of studies improved adherence and only 32% improved health outcomes. They concluded that for long-term treatments, no simple interventions, and only some complex ones, led to improvements in health outcomes. Just 5 of the 93 studies used some form of telehealth, and these could not be aggregated or compared with other methods due to their heterogeneity of modes and clinical settings.

However, some home telehealth trials have included adherence to medication as one of a range of outcomes. In the area of heart failure, two studies have found that home telemonitoring improved the use of beta-blockers [19, 20], although Ramaekers [21] reported no difference in medication adherence, being uniformly high in the telehealth and the control arm of their trial. A trial of home videophones vs telephone or usual care for patients with heart failure found that once a week video communication to reinforce the plan of care did not improve adherence, however, participants were not directly watched taking their medication [22].

2.2 Supporting Cognitively Impaired Clients

New strategies for home delivery of medication management for people with cognitive impairment are needed because the aging population of many developed countries means that the prevalence of dementia will rise. For example, a recent major report in Australia stated that the number of Australians with dementia in 2008 was 230,000, or about 1% of the population, and this is predicted to increase to 730,000, or 2% of the population, by 2050 [23]. Also, the demand for workforce will increase faster than supply, leading to a shortfall of about 59,000 paid staff and 94,000 family carers by 2029. Despite this obvious problem, the strategy and recommendations section of the report makes only a passing mention of telehealth as a possibility for delivering specialist expertise to rural areas [23].

A review of medication management for patients with dementia noted that while reduced cognitive function was a major reason for lack of adherence, this reduction in cognitive function was very often not detected by the treating health care providers [24]. Factors associated with lower adherence are living alone, complex medication regimens, low income, low education, current smoking and problem drinking. Along with all of these factors, the co-existence of depression further reduces adherence. A less expected finding was that being self-reliant and independent reduces adherence, and having greater impairment increases adherence, which is the opposite of what one would expect in people who do not have cognitive impairment, but the authors propose that the reason for this is that independently-minded people with dementia are less likely to accept support [24]. This review also mentioned telehealth only as a future possibility.

However, in considering possible strategies, telehealth was seen by RDNS SA as a potentially valuable solution, since as well as its uses in cognitive assessment at a distance [25, 26], telehealth has also been used for dementia management [27] and to support family carers [28].

2.3 Directly Observed Therapy for Tuberculosis

Tuberculosis (TB) is an infectious disease that needs several months of antibiotic treatment, hence the risk of non-adherence is high. Failure to complete treatment leads to prolonged infectiousness of the individual and the development of drug-resistant TB, which is a public health risk [29]. To overcome these problems, the World Health Organisation has recommended TB patients have Directly Observed Therapy (DOT), that is, are watched taking their tablets, as part of an improved system of TB control [30]. The need for direct observation has been controversial because three systematic reviews have concluded that there is no difference in TB cure rates between DOT and non-DOT treatment programs [29, 31, 32]. However, when the individual studies that contributed to these reviews are looked at, the completion rates of DOT are poor. This might be expected in developing countries due to pressure on health services, but this is also the case for studies from the US and Canada, where completion rates ranged from 20 to 66% [29]. An RCT in Australia trained family members to deliver DOT, because they said daily observation by nurses was extremely expensive, and found no difference between DOT and self-administration, but one-third of the sample could not have DOT because they lived alone, and the overall level of non-compliance in the remainder was 24% [33]. In addition, qualitative research has found that adherence to DOT is reduced because people with TB feel stigmatised, and DOT services often do not fit into people's schedules, making it hard to combine work with treatment, or to maintain confidentiality [34]. In summary, the previous research gives a picture of DOT not being optimally implemented because of practical and social difficulties.

Home videophones are an alternative method for delivering DOT, which offer greater convenience and privacy for clients. There were two DOT clients in the pilot study to this service [1], and a small scale study was conducted in the US with 6 TB clients, which showed that home videophones were a feasible and cost-effective alternative to in-person observation [35]. RDNS SA had been operating a DOT service by home visits, and found difficulties with clients feeling stigmatized, and not being home to receive the visits. Therefore, only some of the medication observations were taking place. In particular, many of the DOT clients were young, had English as a second language and were not inclined to wait at home for a face-to-face visit from a nurse to observe medication administration.

2.4 Innovative Elements of the Project

A number of innovations in both the clinical and the technical services were necessary for this project to advance beyond the trial phase.

2.4.1 Home Videophones in Medication Management

This is the first project that has developed medication management with home videophones beyond a small-scale pilot study. Videophones were chosen as the mode of delivery, because they look like and operate like regular telephones. This makes them particularly suited to home care, because people with no IT skills or experience can use them, nor does the client require a home computer. This is important because the home care clients are most often older with limited incomes, and the very few who had home computers were unable to operate them effectively. Therefore, using videoconferencing software was not an option.

While much of the home telehealth reported in the literature uses monitoring with data transmission, real-time video communication to the home has been used in areas such as post-operative follow-up [36], acute medical treatment [37], palliative care [38], and to help older people stay at home longer [39]. A systematic review of economic analyses of video communication in telehealth found that home care was the area where the greatest cost-effectiveness could be demonstrated [40].

Trials and feasibility studies of home videophones with older people have found that people with cognitive impairment can use videophones. Poon [41] showed that community-dwelling older persons with mild dementia could be assessed and given cognitive intervention via videophone, and that this led to an improvement in their functioning. Savenstedt [42–44] has looked in detail at how older people with cognitive impairment respond to videophone communication, and has found that this particular form of communication can increase the attentiveness and focus of this group. Mochizuki-Kawai [45] reported an apparent increase in verbal fluency after videophone conversations with older nursing home residents, including those with dementia, compared to in-person conversations, and hypothesise that this induces an orientation response and reduces distractions.

There have been two pilot studies on the use of videophones in home-based medication management for people with cognitive impairment: one is the pilot study to the RDNS SA service described in this chapter [1], and the other study was conducted in the US by Smith [46], with 8 people who lived alone and had mild dementia. They found that medication compliance was 81% and remained stable in the videophone group, whereas in the control group, compliance fell from 75 to 62% over a 6 month period. Both of these studies found that some episodes of medication management were missed because the clients had either turned off their videophones or had gone out unexpectedly. In the case of the RDNS SA service, an inability to make video contact could be backed up by a field nurse driving to the patient's home for an in-person visit [1].

2.4.2 New Protocols and Procedures

From the beginning of the trial, it was recognised that nursing protocols would need to be adapted from the field nurse service to the telehealth setting, and some new procedures developed to ensure that virtual visits could be delivered safely to appropriate clients.

Eligibility Assessment and Procedures

A set of criteria were developed and refined over time, to select clients who would be suitable for the telehealth service, and currently they are that the client:

1. Requires at least daily administration of medication
2. Has enough understanding of the English language to understand and to be understood
3. Is able to follow verbal directions given in English
4. Does not have a hearing or visual impairment to the extent that it would make it unsafe for them to use telehealth strategies
5. Is able to locate and use the videophone
6. Does not have a history that would predict that they (or someone in the home) would cause damage to the equipment
7. Does not have a history that would predict that they (or someone in the home) would misuse or abuse the RDNS-owned Internet connection or account
8. Has the functional dexterity necessary to extract medications from a sealed dose administration aide, namely a Webster pack

9. Has the ability to develop and follow a routine

10. The client or their Guardian has the ability to provide informed consent.

These criteria were disseminated to the Healthcare Team Leaders and Clinical Service Coordinators. This was supported by telehealth presentations to healthcare staff by the project nurse and Clinical Business Leader at divisional meetings. It was the responsibility of the regular field nurse to determine eligibility for admission to the telehealth program by verifying that the clients met each of the criteria.

Suitability Assessment and Procedures

Once it has been determined that the client is eligible for the service, the next step is an in-home suitability assessment with a senior nurse. This assessment includes:

1. A functional assessment of the client's ability to consistently:

   a. locate the telephone
   b. respond appropriately and with reasonable confidence to 'over-the-phone' requests, directions and instructions
   c. locate the medication
   d. reliably remove all medications for the required day and time,

2. An environmental assessment to identify:

   a. the most appropriate place to set up the phone and modem including any factors that may contribute to increasing the risk to the client
   b. whether a or not medication administration aid such as a Webster pack is in place and, if not, obtain the client's/carer's consent to organize a pack to be delivered
   c. that oral medication could only be administered when prompted from a sealed dose administration aid

2.4.3 Solving Connectivity Problems

The third innovative element involved solving connectivity problems for real time video to the home, because obtaining adequate bandwidth is a significant issue. It is possible to operate videophones over the PSTN (Public Switched Telephone Network), which is the standard copper wire domestic landline, but the low bandwidth gives a reduced quality, jerky image with a frame rate of 2–3 per second. Previous studies have shown that homecare can be provided effectively using the PSTN [36, 37, 47–49], and the Veteran's Health Administration in the US has made extensive use of PSTN videophones [50]. However, for the particular purpose of medication management, a sharper picture and higher frame rate, of 12–15 per second, is needed to give a smooth, clear image of the person taking or injecting their medication.

For the RNDS SA pilot study, broadband DSL was installed in clients homes [1], and the Smith study used ISDN, or digital telephone lines, to the home [46].

However, for the RDNS SA service, the initial approach of utilising DSL was not ideal: firstly broadband was not available to all homes, because some types of copper wire connections do not support DSL, and also some local telephone exchanges had no spare broadband capacity. Secondly, even where broadband was available, it was not always suitable, because the service needed to be of high reliability with minimal downtime, and to have an upload and download speed of at least 384 kbits/s. Download speed was not a problem, but sourcing sufficient upload speed was sometimes difficult. Thirdly, there was a 1–3 week wait for broadband installation, and this caused delays and dropouts in recruiting clients to the service.

Therefore the RDNS SA worked with a small technology company to develop an entirely new system of connectivity to run the service. In brief, the home videophones were configured to operate through the mobile data network, also known as 3G. This meant that installation could be done with just a power supply, and worked well provided that the appropriate router and antenna were installed with the videophone. Generally an antenna inside the house, next to the video-phone, was all that was needed, but in one or two cases a roof mounting was required. This original approach has allowed installations to proceed with much greater speed and flexibility.

3 Outcome of the Project

The outcome of the project resulted in the initial trial becoming a medium scale, ongoing service, and this is significant because the translation of telehealth into sustainable operations is a well known problem in the field, with reviews noting that surprisingly few telehealth applications proceeded beyond the research and development phase [51]. Combining a number of studies into telehealth translation shows that there are a group of factors associated with successful introduction into routine care [51–54]: that the telehealth service solves local problems, whether these be medical, political or of service delivery, that there is a high degree of collaboration with external partners, that the internal organizational, financial and technical problems are addressed, that systematic planning involving all who are affected takes place, and that a degree of integration can be achieved. Integration can be a vague concept, but Atun supplies an operational definition; that integration has occurred when governance, funding, planning, monitoring, evaluation and demand generation for the service are all carried out by the same mechanisms as for the general service delivery of the organisation [55, 56]. Using these criteria, the RDNS SA service has achieved integration.

Introducing a telehealth service into a healthcare organization is a complex innovation, because it requires changes to existing professional roles and work practices, as well as needing to be adapted to local conditions [57]. In seeking to understand how best to guide such a complex innovation into normal operations, the well known diffusion model of Rogers, which has become a dominant paradigm of the innovation field [58], does not provide all the answers. May studied the implementation of a telepsychiatry service and concluded that a linear model of diffusion could not account for the normalisation outcomes, which were more determined by political, organisational and ownership issues [59]. He went on to develop a theory called the normalisation process model, in which the key elements are what can be dealt with in each consultation or other interaction of the service (interactional workability), how the new service relates to existing knowledge in the organisation (relational integration), how division of labour is accomplished (skill set workability), and how resource allocation and governance are achieved (contextual integration) [60]. This model has the advantage of being relevant to a planned introduction of a new service into a structured setting.

The normalisation process model has proved to be useful for understanding the success of this project, because each of its components has been applicable to the implementation processes. The elements of the home visit for medication management have been carefully redefined for the telehealth environment, and new interaction elements, for example the client's ability to initiate a call to the service, have been purposefully introduced. The existing knowledge and culture of the organisation was assessed, and an explicit change management strategy, supported by senior management, and described in the next section, was conducted. The management tasks of allocation of labour and resources were also closely attended to, and were aided by the existence of a call centre which has a very close relationship with the field service, so new communication links were not needed; indeed, many of the nurses in the call centre had previously worked in the field service. Lastly, changes to finance and staff reporting arrangements could be readily accomplished by existing processes.

4 Internal Influences on Development and Outcome

Within the RDNS SA, existing organisational structures and culture influenced the project, therefore a change management strategy was implemented to ensure that development proceeded as smoothly as possible.

4.1 Case-Finding and Referrals

RDNS SA field services nurses were expected to find and refer suitable clients for the videophone service. As part of usual operations, the teams of field nurses discuss, on a daily basis, their capacity to manage the workload, and the intention was to introduce assessing eligibility for telehealth into this existing work process. Suitable clients typically had between 2 and 3 in-home visits per day, hence it was felt that identifying them for the videophone service would be a motivator, because this would provide the field teams with much needed additional capacity for in-home visits.

However nurses did not immediately or routinely 'case find' clients appropriate for the videophone service. In order to bring the videophone service into 'business as usual' a dedicated senior nurse worked with home visiting staff. Early in this process it was found that the assessment tools used to determine if a patient was suitable for videophone services needed to be refined. The nurses concerned also lacked the experience in how to teach an adult with cognitive impartment how to use the technology.

4.2 Education for Change

A senior nurse went to staff meetings and team meetings and presented the updated admission assessment tool to staff, who were then able to ask questions and receive answers to any clinical concerns that they had. These face-to-face discussions, which allowed honest and open debate regarding the clinical efficacy of this new service was critical in gaining overall acceptance.

Some staff were suspicious of the program and saw it as a measure aimed only at cutting costs, so it was essential that these concerns were addressed. Two approaches were taken: firstly a cogent rationale was presented as to why this innovation was required within the business. Population statistics demonstrating the ageing population and increasing rates of dementia were effectively used to show that with people on videophone programs, it would allow the organization to see more clients for the same cost. The second important message to discuss with staff was feedback from the clients themselves, which is discussed further below. Some clients expressed their gratitude in not having a nurse enter their home on a daily basis; they stated it was less invasive and therefore a more acceptable form of service delivery for some people. The DOT clients in particular, were very positive because they could arrange their virtual visits around their work schedules. Conveying this message allowed the expression of an alternative to the dominant view that all people preferred a home visit, which has proved to be a myth that was not truly based on client feedback.

5 External Influences on Development and Outcome

External influences had less influence than one might expect on this project, because the RDNS SA is a larger sized community nursing organisation, and was capable of developing the telehealth service within its usual operations. Legal and professional indemnity issues were considered and it was found that existing arrangements were adequate. As the service was operated wholly within the jurisdiction of South Australia, professional registration was also not a problem. Additionally, the services are provided for the usual urban area of RDNS SA operations, so there was no need to negotiate with providers from other regions. Nonetheless, the following external factors were significant:

5.1 Economic Aspects

Economic aspects made an impact on the decision to expand and continue the service. Comparative analysis of cost clearly indicates that this telehealth service has a distinct advantage over the traditional field nurse service delivery model, saving approximately $1,400 per client per year (based on two medication visits seven days per week). Telehealth for this client group is thus a viable cost-effective strategy, and allows efficiencies to be made in the distribution of the nursing workforce.

5.2 Medical Practitioners

The clients' usual general medical practitioner (GP), is clearly an important partner in the treating team, and the GP is informed about the intention to bring the client into the telehealth service, with the opportunity to raise any concerns, or request that the client not be managed by telehealth. The vast majority of GPs have been positive and supportive of the service. There is an obvious future possibility for general medical practices to join the videophone network and also do virtual home visits, but this has not happened to date. It is likely that the main reasons for this are:

1. As the 73 clients on the videophone services are scattered over the metropolitan area, no single general practice is caring for more than a few clients each.
2. The Australian universal health insurance scheme only reimburse GPs for work done face-to-face, so the absence of payment for tele-consultations is a disincentive.

5.3 Government Relations

The major funders of the care provided by the RDNS SA are the South Australian state government, and the federal government of Australia, who provide the funding for packages of care to be delivered to individual clients, therefore it was necessary to inform both governments of the intention to develop a telehealth option for some clients. Meetings were held and resulted in approval to use the videophone service without changing current funding arrangements.

6 User Aspects

To assist in the evaluation of this new service ten interviews were conducted with people who were living with a chronic illness or condition and were using tele-health services for medication administration. All were adults, aged 18 years or over, and most had been using the videophone for a period of 3–4 months. The aim of the interviews was to explore the client's experiences of receiving healthcare from RDNS nurses via the videophone.

6.1 Thematic Analysis of Evaluation

Five major themes were identified following analysis of interview data. These were:

1. Improved health as an outcome of receiving medication reminders via the videophone
2. Confidence and reassurance as a consequence of using the videophone
3. The importance of continuity with nurses
4. The videophone reduces the intrusion of healthcare
5. Ease of use

Detailed examination of these themes gives the following results, supplemented by typical examples within each theme.

6.1.1 Improved Health Outcomes

All participants reported observable improvements in their health as a direct result of receiving medication reminders on the videophone. Physical, psychological and social improvements also impacted on their health. For example, participant E described positive changes in his outlook and stabilisation of his epilepsy:

> I've found it 100% successful... I find that since I am being closely monitored and taking my medication on cue I don't have anywhere near as many seizures. In fact I don't have any ... I find that now I'm interested in meeting people and getting along with people... I used to sit around drinking [alcohol] a lot and worrying about having seizures. I don't do that anymore.

Participant G's son noticed that his mother's chronic conditions have stabilised since she has used the videophone:

> I know from taking mum to the doctor's appointment I have noticed that since she's been taking tablets regular and the timing of her tablets [has been correct]... it has leveled out all of her conditions, the diabetes, blood pressure...they are back on track!

He goes on to describe the benefits of contact for his mother who would otherwise be alone much of the time:

Mum does have some significant health issues and given her age [82]... I just think that it's good that she has that regular contact. It makes it a bit easier for me too... to know she hasn't fallen in the middle of night... it's [RDNS] a fantastic service.

6.1.2 Confidence and Reassurance

Some participants experienced an increase in confidence knowing they could use the videophone to call the nurse, and access assistance any time. Participant B describes how it has helped her to take medication on time, and reduce anxiety related to the medication:

> ... the main benefit is that you <u>have</u> to take the medication. I used to forget it and I used to argue with mum... they call you on the videophone and if you don't answer they call you on the mobile so you have to take it. ... [The nurses] are so caring... most of them ask about me ...they tell me 'don't worry the medication is alright' ... and it makes me feel good

Participant F explains how the videophone gives comfort to both his family and himself after having a major health crisis:

> ...it is a comfort for my family just knowing there somebody there in case I need to... if there's an issue. And I know they are there ... it's important especially to someone like me who thought I had a mild heart attack and it damn near killed me.

6.1.3 The Importance of Continuity with Nurses

The telehealth service has greater continuity of care than the field service, and all participants valued having the same few nurses at the end of the videophone. This contributed to familiarity and trust between the nurse and client, and was especially important for those with memory or hearing impairment. Participant F, who has memory loss, said:

> Yes it gives me confidence to have the same nurses...I'm still dealing with the memory loss so having things that are the same [is important]... I have this memory loss ... so I don't want to pick up the phone and speak to a different person.

Participant H's response is typical of others as she states:

> ... it's rarely that I have a new nurse and it's nice having the same nurses.

6.1.4 The Videophone Reduces the Intrusion of Healthcare

All participants expressed a strong preference for their healthcare to be delivered via the videophone rather than a home visit. This was an unexpected finding, and the reasons given included convenience, less intrusion, and flexibility. While it might be assumed that receiving healthcare via the videophone may impair the relationship between the nurse and client this did not appear to be the case. Participant G explains:

> ... there's not much difference between the videophone and a home visit... the relationship with the nurses is similar.

Three participants said they preferred the videophone because they were able to carry on with their life without the restriction of waiting at home for the nurse to visit. Participant D said:

> ... it's definitely better having a home visit... I may not be home when they call and this way I can ring them if I'm going out.

Participant G talks about the reasons why he prefers the videophone for his mother:

> ... I think the big thing is the regularity and the timing of the calls... I think that they call in about nine o'clock every day... it's really good... [with home visits] if the nursing staff gets stuck at a house it can be a couple of hours later and it holds mum up from going out or whatever...

Participant F said that he received more time with the nurse on the phone than he does during a home visit:

> I think I get a better service with the videophone because I know when they are going to call. With the nurse visits they are always time poor so I'd get more time on the phone.

Participant F explained that the videophone is less intrusive:

> I feel good about it [the videophone]. [With the home visits] my biggest fear was that I'd have strangers walking in and out of the house every day and I didn't like the thought of that.

6.1.5 Ease of Use

Most clients found the videophone easy to use, comparing it to the use of a normal telephone. Two clients were concerned about their ability to master the technology, and three were worried about how it would fit with their busy lifestyle. However, it soon became apparent to all that there would not be any problems. Participant A said:

> I was worried because maybe you [RDNS] would call me and I would not be home. I am new to this country and I am very busy... I have lots of appointments and I thought maybe I'd be wasting your [RDNS] time. [I worried that] they will call and I am not home. But actually I have adapted and it works much better than that...

Participant H was hesitant initially but soon realised she could manage it:

> ...at first I dreaded it [learning to use the videophone]...beforehand not being put through the paces... not knowing... I thought 'oh dear, what am I going to do'... I thought I wouldn't understand but as you know there's nothing to it.

However participant F would have preferred to have more information at the beginning:

> Initially it felt quite demeaning for quite some time…the fact that it has to be a Webster pack…that's added cost and it means I have less control over my prescriptions…I've always been in control of my life. Perhaps in the introduction you could explain that a little better … I'd spend a bit more time before you set it up… explaining the details… this is what you do and the reason we do this is to guarantee you don't make a mistake with the tablets.

6.2 Summary of User Experiences

The experience of using the videophone was deemed as positive for all participants. There is a direct association between using the videophone for medication reminders and an improvement in the timing and regularity of taking medication. This has resulted in positive health outcomes with participants feeling better from a stabilisation of the chronic illness or condition they live with. Interestingly this appears to have had a 'snowball' effect of increasing confidence, feelings of security and interest in life for some clients. Most participants found learning to use the videophone easy. The few that had initial concerns soon discovered they had mastered it successfully. All participants preferred the videophone to a home visit, considering it to be a less intrusive way to receive healthcare. The benefit of being able to contact the nurse via the videophone was valued by most participants, providing reassurance and confidence. Clearly this has been a very successful strategy for delivering health care to people living with chronic illness or conditions in their homes in the community.

7 General Aspects

Evaluation of the telehealth service also produced information about these general effects of the project:

7.1 Safety Outcomes

According to the telehealth participants who were interviewed the technology was very reliable and safe, with the videophone exchange being available almost 100% of the time. Technical assistance was rated as excellent, with minor issues being resolved quickly, within 24 h. There was a significant reduction in the reporting of medication errors or mishaps. The severity score for all but one of these incidents was assessed as either minor or insignificant. The incidents with medications that were reported provide insights that may need to be considered during the assessment and setting up phase. One error was due to a lack of communication between health care services, one was the result of clients receiving inappropriate additional medication instructions from a pharmacy delivery person, another could be attributed to the client adjusting to the process of receiving medications via the videophone, and two incidents related to behavioural and cognitive issues characteristic of people living with cognitive impairment. These clients received a home visit that resulted in reassessment for suitability to the program.

7.2 Clinical Outcomes

A significant finding of this research is that receiving support with medications via telehealth appears to have the effect of stabilising participant's health conditions resulting in them experiencing well-being and improved quality of health. The findings of the interviews conducted with ten participants suggests that this is directly associated with increased compliance with medications and/or treatment. Interviews with participants revealed that additional benefits were experienced including increased self-confidence, an increased sense of security and for some, reduced isolation. These psychosocial benefits can only contribute to wellbeing.

7.3 Medication Management Outcomes

There are indications that some clients increased their ability to manage their medication as a result of being prompted by the videophone and there was evidence of some clients taking responsibility for remembering medications without prompting or supervision. Participants who were interviewed reported an increased awareness of the need to take medication at the right time and a willingness to be responsible for taking it. Some clients had their medication ready in preparation for the phone call. Not only did clients take their medication regularly and on time but also those with three and four times daily medications were able to receive support via videophone that would not have been possible with home visits.

8 Conclusion

This project has demonstrated that it is possible to set up a successful medication management service in an urban environment, using real time video communication to the home. The service started as a feasibility trial, became an integrated part of community nursing services, and has now been operating for over 3 years. An evaluation of the service indicate that telehealth is a safe, effective, cost saving method of delivering medications to the growing numbers of people living in the community with cognitive impairment, and also offers a way to improve the implementation of Directly Observed Therapy for tuberculosis. The unexpected finding from the evaluation was the preference of many clients for the video option; it proved not to be a second-best option to a face-to-face service, but to have its own unique advantages.

8.1 Research Developments

The literature shows that telehealth has not yet become a mainstream solution to promoting medication adherence. Since medication management is such a large-scale problem, there is an interest and a market for technical innovations, resulting in a plethora of systems that automate some or all of the medication management process. Examples that are available, or are in the research and development phase include:

A combination of medication bottles with 'smart caps', a dispenser, and a modem that transmits a signal when the bottles are opened, and sends an alarm if adherence falls below 50% [61].

A computer based system that sends patient data automatically to a server, where it is analysed in real time and non-compliance alerts are sent to nurses [62].

A tracking system that uses sensors in the home, and prompts the patient via a 'messaging watch' when they are in the correct context at home to take medication [63].

Robots that move around the person's home providing adherence and appointment reminders [64], or containing a medication dispenser [65].

An integrated wearable home sensor and feedback system for cardiovascular disease [66].

8.2 Acceptability and Usability Issues

In theory, a fully automated system could replace a system using home visits or real-time video, and further reduce the health workforce needed to monitor the chronically unwell. However, a cautionary note is sounded by a study with older veterans, that tested the functionality and usability of a range of medication management devices that are available on the market today, and found that patients were unwilling to pay and unlikely to use them. An additional problem noted was that many devices ran on batteries so there is a danger that patients would let them go flat. Also, the manufacturers' instructions were inadequate and inconsistent, and needed to be rewritten by the researchers before they could be understood by participants [67]. Another study used a medication box which transmitted data to an electronic health record each time it was opened, and half the study population did not want to continue using it, reporting that they did not want to be observed in their daily living [68]. A sample of patients who reported forgetting to take anti-depressants were asked if they would be willing to receive text message reminders; 59% agreed and 41% refused [69]. This method would be less useful in the older population as there are lower levels of mobile phone use, and cognitively impaired people are usually unable to manage a mobile phone, particularly text messaging.

8.3 Future Possibilities

While real time video is the mainstay of this home telehealth service, there is a possibility of adopting other technical innovations, such as those described above.

However, much work remains to be done in translating these developments into scaled up, workable systems that can be shown to deliver improvements to routine care. It may be that a multi-modal system could be the most useful option, with some clients able and willing to use a more automated approach, but those with greater impairment, social/emotional difficulties, or a public health requirement for direct observation, needing a real person on the other end of the screen. Telehealth offers RDNS SA and its clients numerous exciting opportunities both now and in the near future. It builds on the RDNS SA stated aim of "the right people in the right place, with the right attitude and skills, doing the right thing at the right time".

References

1. Wade V, Izzo J, Hamlyn J. Videophone delivery of medication management in community nursing. e-J Health Inform. 2009;4:e1
2. Botsis T, Hartvigsen G. Current status and future perspectives in telecare for elderly people suffering from chronic diseases. J Telemed Telecare. 2008;14:195–203.
3. Martinez A, Everss E, Rojo-Alvarez JL, Figal DP, Garcia-Alberola A. A systematic review of the literature on home monitoring for patients with heart failure. J Telemed Telecare. 2006;12:234–41.
4. Barlow J, Singh D, Bayer S, Curry R. A systematic review of the benefits of home telecare for frail elderly people and those with long-term conditions. J Telemed Telecare. 2007;13:172–9.
5. Gaikwad R, Warren J. The role of home-based information and communications technology interventions in chronic disease management: a systematic review. Health Inform J. 2009;15:122–36.
6. Pare G, Moquadem K, Pineau G, St-Hilaire C. Clinical effects of home telemonitoring in the context of diabetes, asthma, heart failure and hypertension: a systematic review. J Med Internet Res. 2010;12:e21.
7. Osterberg L, Blascheke T. Adherence to medication. N Engl J Med. 2005;353:487–97.
8. Feldman PH, Totten AM, Foust J, Naik D, Costello B, Kurtzman E, McDonald M. Medication management: evidence brief. Center for home care policy & research. Home Healthc Nurse. 2009;27:379–86.
9. Cooper J, Hall L, Penland A, Krueger A, May J. Measuring medication adherence. Popul Health Manag. 2009;12:25–30.

10. Larsen J, Stovring H, Kragstrup J, Hansen DG. Can differences in medical drug compliance between European countries be explained by social factors: analyses based on data from the European Social Survey, round 2. BMC Public Health. 2009;9:145.
11. van Dulmen S, Slujis E, van Dijk L, de Ridder D, Heerdink R, Bensing J. Patient adherence to medical treatment: a review of reviews. BMC Health Serv Res. 2007;7:55.
12. S. a. Q. Council. Second national report on patient safety: improving medication safety. Canberra: Commonwealth Department of Health and Aging; 2002.
13. Kuzuya M, Hirakawa Y, Suzuki Y, Iwata M, Enoki H, Hasegawa J, Iguchi A. Association between unmet needs for medication support and all-cause hospitalization in community-dwelling disabled elderly people. J Am Geriatr Soc. 2008;56:881–6.
14. Shearer J. Improving oral medication management in home health agencies. Home Healthc Nurse. 2009;27:184–92.
15. Mager DD, Madigan EA. Medication use among older adults in a home care setting. Home Healthc Nurse. 2010;28:14–21.
16. Cooper C, Carpenter I, Katona C, Schroll M, Wagner C, Fialova D, Livingston G. The AdHOC study of older adults' adherence to medication in 11 countries. Am J Geriatr Psychiatry. 2005;13:1067–76.
17. Stafford AC, Tenni PC, Peterson GM, Jackson SL, Hejlesen A, Villesen C, Rasmussen M. Drug-related problems identified in medication reviews by Australian pharmacists. Pharm World Sci. 2009;31:216–23.
18. Haynes RB, Ackloo E, Sahota N, McDonald HP, Yao X. Interventions for enhancing medication adherence. In: Cochrane Database Syst Rev: John Wiley & Sons, Ltd.; 2008.
19. Antonicelli R, Testarmata P, Spazzafumo L, Gagliardi C, Bilo G, Valentini M, Olivieri F, Parati G. Impact of telemonitoring at home on the management of elderly patients with congestive heart failure. J Telemed Telecare. 2008;14:300–5.
20. Cleland JGF, Louis AA, Rigby AS, Janssens U, Balk AH. Noninvasive home telemonitoring for patients with heart failure at high risk of recurrent admision and death. J Am Coll Cardiol. 2005;45:1654–64.
21. Ramaekers BL, Janssen-Boyne JJ, Gorgels AP, Vrijhoef HJ. Adherence among telemonitored patients with heart failure to pharmacological and nonpharmacological recommendations. Telemed J E Health. 2009;15:517–24.
22. Wakefield BJ, Holman JE, Ray A, Scherubel M, Burns TL, Kienzle MG, Rosenthal GE. Outcomes of a home telehealth intervention for patients with heart failure. J Telemed Telecare. 2009;15:46–50.
23. Access Economics Pty Ltd. Making choices: Future dementia care: projections, problems and preferences.http://www.accesseconomics.com.au/publicationsreports/showreport.php?id=196 2009; Accessed 14 April 2011.
24. Arlt S, Lindner R, Rosler A, von Renteln-Kruse W. Adherence to medication in patients with dementia: predictors and strategies for improvement. Drugs Ag. 2008;25:1033–47.
25. Saligari J, Flicker L, Loh PK, Maher S, Ramesh P, Goldswain P. The clinical achievements of a geriatric telehealth project in its first year. J Telemed Telecare. 2002;8(S3):53–5.
26. Shores MM, Ryan-Dykes P, Williams RM, Mamerto B, Sadak T, Pascualy M, Felker BL, Zweigle M, Nichol P, Peskind ER. Identifying undiagnosed dementia in residential care veterans: comparing telemedicine to in-person clinical examination. Int J Geriatr Psychiatry. 2004;19:101–8.
27. Morgan DG, Crossley M, Kirk A, D'Arcy C, Stewart N, Biem J, Forbes D, Harder S, Basran J, Dal Bello-Haas V, McBain L. Improving access to dementia care: development and evaluation of a rural and remote memory clinic. Aging Ment Health. 2009;13:17–30.
28. Powell J, Chiu T, Eysenbach G. A systematic review of networked technologies supporting carers of people with dementia. J Telemed Telecare. 2008;14:154–6.
29. Hirsch-Moverman Y, Daftary A, Franks J, Colson PW. Adherence to treatment for latent tuberculosis infection: systematic review of studies in the US and Canada. Int J Tuberc Lung Dis. 2008;12:1235–54.

30. World Health Organisation, "WHO Report 2009 Global tuberculosis control," World Health Organisation 2009, Geneva.
31. Volmink J, Garner P. Directly observed therapy for treating tuberculosis. *Cochrane Database Syst Rev*. 2007. p. CD003343.
32. Kruk ME, Schwalbe NR, Aguiar CA. Timing of default from tuberculosis treatment: a systematic review. Trop Med Int Health. 2008;13:703–12.
33. MacIntyre CR, Goebel K, Brown GV, Skull S, Starr M, Fullinfaw RO. A randomised controlled clinical trial of the efficacy of family-based direct observation of anti-tuberculosis treatment in an urban, developed-country setting. Int J Tuberc Lung Dis. 2003;7:848–54.
34. Noyes J, Popay J. Directly observed therapy and tuberculosis: how can a systematic review of qualitative research contribute to improving services? A qualitative meta-synthesis. J Adv Nurs. 2007;57:227–43.
35. DeMaio J, Schwartz L, Cooley P, Tice A. The application of telemedicine technology to a directly observed therapy program for tuberculosis: a pilot project. Clin Infect Dis. 2001;33:2082–4.
36. Bohnenkamp SK, McDonald P, Lopez AM, Krupinski E, Blackett A. Traditional versus telenursing outpatient management of patients with cancer with new ostomies. Oncol Nurs Forum. 2004;31:1005–10.
37. Eron L, Marineau M. Telemedicine: treating infections in the home. Infect Med. 2006;23:517.
38. Bensink ME, Armfield NR, Pinkerton R, Irving H, Hallahan AR, Theodoros DG, Russell T, Barnett AG, Scuffham PA, Wootton R. Using videotelephony to support paediatric oncology-related palliative care in the home: from abandoned RCT to acceptability study. Palliat Med. 2009;23:228–37.
39. Croghan JE, Prince TR, Zekic L, Underwood J, Sheridan PH Jr, Weatherly J, Knohl K. Comprehensive approach to automated assistive telemanagement for seniors in their home or residence-pilot program results. J Ambul Care Manage. 2007;30:318–26.
40. Wade VA, Karnon J, Elshaug AE, Hiller JE. A systematic review of economic analyses of telehealth services using real time video communication. BMC Health Serv Res. 2010;10:233.
41. Poon P, Hui E, Dai D, Kwok T, Woo J. Cognitive intervention for community-dwelling older persons with memory problems: telemedicine versus face-to-face treatment. Int J Geriatr Psychiatry. 2005;20:285–6.
42. Savenstedt S, Zingmark K, Sandman PO. Video-phone communication with cognitively impaired elderly patients. J Telemed Telecare. 2003;9(S2):52–4.
43. Savenstedt S, Brulin C, Sandman PO. Family members' narrated experiences of communicating via video-phone with patients with dementia staying at a nursing home. J Telemed Telecare. 2003;9:216–20.
44. Savenstedt S, Zingmark K, Hyden LC, Brulin C. Establishing joint attention in remote talks with the elderly about health: a study of nurses' conversation with elderly persons in teleconsultations. Scand J Caring Sci. 2005;19:317–24.
45. Mochizuki-Kawai H, Tanaka M, Suzuki T, Yamakawa Y, Mochizuki S, Arai M, Kawamura M. Elderly adults improve verbal fluency by videophone conversations: a pilot study. J Telemed Telecare. 2008;14:215–8.
46. Smith GE, Lunde AM, Hathaway JC, Vickers KS. Telehealth home monitoring of solitary persons with mild dementia. Am J Alzheimers Dis Other Demen. 2007;22:20–6.
47. Finkelstein SM, Speedie SM, Potthoff S. Home telehealth improves clinical outcomes at lower cost for home healthcare. Telemed J E Health. 2006;12:128–36.
48. Jerant AF, Azari R, Nesbitt TS. Reducing the cost of frequent hospital admissions for congestive heart failure: a randomized trial of a home telecare intervention. Med Care. 2001;39:1234–45.
49. Smith RV. The digital camera in clinical practice. Otolaryngol Clin North Am. 2002;35:1175–89.

50. Darkins A, Ryan P, Kobb R, Foster L, Edmonson E, Wakefield B, Lancaster AE. Care coordination/Home telehealth: the systematic implementation of health informatics, home telehealth, and disease management to support the care of veteran patients with chronic conditions. Telemed J E Health. 2008;14:1118–26.
51. Obstfelder A, Engeseth K, Wynn R. Characteristics of successfully implemented telemedical applications. Implemen Sci. 2007;2:25
52. Barlow J, Bayer S, Curry R. The design of pilot telecare projects and their integration into mainstream service delivery. J Telemed Telecare. 2003;9(S1):1–3.
53. Aas IHM. "The organizational challenge for health care from telemedicine and e-health,". Oslo: Work Res Inst; 2007.
54. Broens TH, Huis in't Veld RM, Vollenbroek-Hutten MM, Hermens HJ, van Halteren AT, Nieuwenhuis LJ. Determinants of successful telemedicine implementations: a literature study. J Telemed Telecare. 2007;13:303–9.
55. Atun R, de Jongh T, Secci F, Ohiri K, Adeyi O. A systematic review of the evidence on integration of targeted health interventions into health systems. Health Policy Plan. 2010;25:1–14.
56. Atun R, de Jongh T, Secci F, Ohiri K, Adeyi O. Integration of targeted health interventions into health systems: a conceptual framework for analysis. Health Policy Plan. 2010;25:104–11.
57. Plesk P. Complexity and the adoption of innovation in health care. Washington, DC: National Institute for Health Care Management Foundation; 2003.
58. Estabrooks CA, Derksen L, Winther C, Lavis JN, Scott SD, Wallin L, Prefetto-McGrath J. The intellectual structure, substance of the knowledge utilisation field: a longitudinal author co-citation analysis, 1945 to 2004. Implement Sci. 2008;3:49.
59. May C, Harrison R, Finch T, MacFarlane A, Mair FS, Wallace P. Understanding the normalisation of telemedicine services through qualitative evaluation. J Am Med Inform Assoc. 2003;10:596–604.
60. May C. A rational model for assessing and exaluating complex interventions in health care. BMC Health Serv Res. 2006;6:86.
61. Frangou S, Sachpazidis I, Stassinakis A, Sakas G. Telemonitoring of medication adherence in patients with schizophrenia. Telemed J E Health. 2005;11:675–83.
62. Finkelstein J, Cha E. Hypertension telemanagement in blacks. Circ Cardiovasc Qual Outcomes. 2009;2:272–8.
63. Hayes TL, Cobbinah K, Dishongh T, Kaye JA, Kimel J, Labhard M, Leen T, Lundell J, Ozertem U, Pavel M, Philipose M, Rhodes K, Vurgun S. A study of medication-taking and unobtrusive, intelligent reminding. Telemed J E Health. 2009;15:770–6.
64. Oddsson LI, Radomski MV, White M, Nilsson D. A robotic home telehealth platform system for treatment adherence, social assistance and companionship - an overview. Conf Proc IEEE Eng Med Biol Soc. 2009;2009:6437–40.
65. Takacs B, Hanak D. A prototype home robot with an ambient facial interface to improve drug compliance. J Telemed Telecare. 2008;14:393–5.
66. Reiter H, Maglaveras N. Heart Cycle: compliance and effectiveness in HF and CAD closed-loop management. Conf Proc IEEE Eng Med Biol Soc. 2009;2009:299–302.
67. Wakefield BJ, Orris LJ, Holman JE, Russell CL. User perceptions of in-home medication dispensing devices. J Gerontol Nurs. 2008;34:15–25.
68. Schmidt S, Sheikzadeh S, Beil B, Patten M, Stettin J. Acceptance of telemonitoring to enhance medication compliance in patients with chronic heart failure. Telemed J E Health. 2008;14:426–33.
69. Sahm L, MacCurtain A, Hayden J, Roche C, Richards HL. Electronic reminders to improve medication adherence–are they acceptable to the patient? Pharm World Sci. 2009;31:627–9.

The Introduction of Activity Monitoring as Part of Care Delivery to Independently Living Seniors

Charles G. Willems, Marieke D. Spreeuwenberg, Loek A. van der Heide, Luc P. de Witte and John Rietman

Abstract Demographic trends in southern Netherlands predict an increasing aging population in the coming decade. Since there will not be enough health providers available to meet the growing demand of care of the elderly, there is a need to reorganize the Dutch health care system in a more efficient way. In this process, innovative technologies can play an important role. It is speculated that monitoring daily activities may be an effective way to obtain information on well-being of seniors living independently. Alterations in behavior could then be used to support the organization of care delivery to these persons. Technology has become available commercially by which the activities of the elderly living at home are automatically monitored. In the USA this technology mainly is used to support informal carers in their care after their relatives at a distance. The authors speculated that this technology may also be used as a communication infrastructure that can deliver information to care workers. Moreover, this could enable them to re-organize the process of care delivery in such a way that future challenges are met effectively. They were able to set up a series of projects in which this speculation was substantiated. First of all a small pilot experiment was started to demonstrate that the technology was applicable in the province of Limburg in The Netherlands. Not only the technical feasibility could be demonstrated, also the development of a communication infrastructure in which several (international) organizations, each with specific expertise, was completed successfully. Also at the user level (clients and care workers) evidence was gathered that this approach may deliver an adequate support. Next, a large scale implementation project was

---

C. G. Willems · M. D. Spreeuwenberg · L. A. van der Heide · L. P. de Witte
Zuyd University, P.O. Box 550, 6400 AN Heerlen, The Netherlands
e-mail: c.g.m.h.willems@hszuyd.nl

J. Rietman (⌧)
Proteion Thuis, P.O. box 218, 5800 AE Venray, The Netherlands
e-mail: johnrietman@proteion.nl

Commun Med Care Compunetics (2011) 3: 167–179
DOI: 10.1007/8754_2011_22

Published Online: 19 July 2011

started. In this project the consequences of data delivery by the technology in the work process of care deliverers was investigated. Instructional courses and new care management tools targeted at home-care workers were developed to support the effective use of this infrastructure. In the mean time other care organizations were invited to participate in the projects. At the client level, evidence is gathered to demonstrate the effectiveness of the system. The research and implementation projects are now financed by grants. It is the intention of the care organization involved, to use this infrastructure in a regular way. This means that a structural financial scheme had to be developed. Thus information was gathered to set up a business case for the future use of this technology.The results obtained up to now will be discussed in this chapter.

Keywords Activity monitoring · Care at a distance · Independant living

1 Description of the Project

Demographic trends in Southern Netherlands predict an increasing aging population in the coming decade. Since there will not be enough health providers available to meet the growing demand of care of the elderly, there is a need to reorganize the Dutch health care system in a more efficient way. In this process, innovative technologies can play an important role. It is speculated that monitoring daily activities may be an effective means to obtain information on well-being of senior living independently. Alterations in behavior could then be used to support the organization of care delivery to these persons. Based on this analysis, a research institute located in the province of Limburg set up a collaboration with a homecare organization to perform applied research following the above considerations. The starting question for the development of this project was as follows (January 2007). "Is it possible to use technology at home to support care delivery to elderly persons (frail elderly or persons with dementia) in such a way that these persons are supported to maintain their stage of independent living, whereas in the mean time the care delivery process becomes more sustainable". Orientation in the field of technology applications leaded to the identification of commercially available technology that served the cause. A pilot project was organized to test whether the technology could be used within the framework of Dutch homecare organizations (September 2007). After successful completion, a large-scale implementation project was organized (September 2008). This is accompanied by a research project directed towards the effects at the client level (December 2010) and a business case development at the financial/organizational level (June 2010). Currently, activities are undertaken to enable long-term implementation of the approach as part of routine care support to the elderly persons.

2 Development of the Project

2.1 Relevance and Approach of Activity Monitoring

Research indicates that the ability to perform the activities of daily life (ADL-activities) may change as a consequence of the development of aging diseases. Changes in the performance of instrumental ADL-activities such as telephoning, medication use and performance of transfers, appear to be indicative for an ongoing process of dementia development [1]. Gure [2] indicated that a significant reduction occurs in the performance of dressing, eating and toileting activities as compared to non-demented elderly. These differences can be noted between the different types of dementia. These data imply that the detection of early changes in activity pattern of a person may be an effective tool to indicate whether care support is needed. The only prerequisite would be that the changes in activity of the person monitored can be detected without interference in the performance of the activity itself. From a technological point of view several approaches have been followed to measure activities patterns. Taken together these are called smart home technologies. In general, they use techniques such as movement detection by infrared sensors, use of electric appliances such as TV, stoves, light, transfers between different spaces etc. Data communication is done by wired communication protocols (Powerline or homebus technology) or by the use of wireless technologies (IR, Bluetooth, Zigbee). Although these approaches are promising, none of them has already been tested to such a level that clinical effectiveness was achieved [3]. Following a systematic approach, Glascock and Kutzik [4] have developed a system that is based on the use of activity monitoring using a small amount of infrared sensors. Furthermore, they have developed algorithms that may detect activity changes indicative for behavior changes in elderly persons, such as meal preparation behavior, sleeping pattern, mobility, etc. Another advantage is that the technology has become commercially available. Taken together this stimulated the authors to initiate a pilot study to investigate whether this technology can be used for the purpose described above.

2.2 Developing a Pilot Using the Technology

The technology used see Fig. 1 consists of several infrared sensors, and a data gathering unit placed at specific locations in the house. The data are transferred through an analogue telecommunication line to a server. At this level calculations are made and the resulting information is given back to the user. This is done by means of an individual web page and in case of a detected emergency situation directly to a care provider. Due to the fact that emergent situations may occur 24 h a day and 7 days a week and the homecare organization is only reachable during business hours, a solution had to be found. The homecare organization had already

Fig. 1 The technology

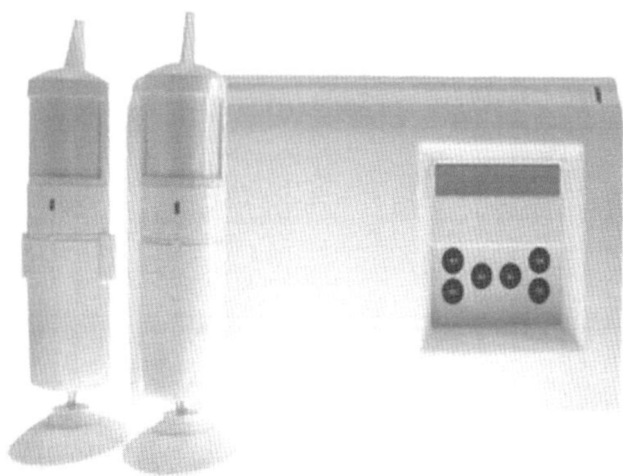

Fig. 2 Scheme of the (data)
communication infrastructure

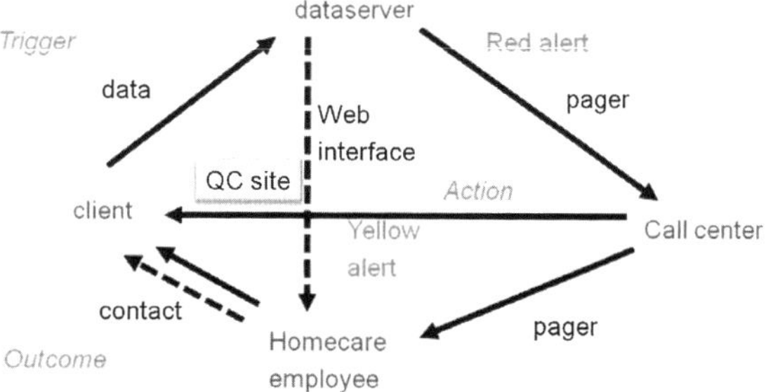

invested in a infrastructure for (the so called) 'unplannable care'. This was
organized by installing a team of care workers that is able to react on short notice.
To guarantee for their reach ability around the clock, they used a call centre to
located at the regional centre for ambulance services. This call centre was used to
receive the urgent messages generated by the technology.

Thus, the resulting data communication infrastructure was set up as presented in
Fig. 2. For each of the steps, a protocol was developed stating the actions that have
to be taken in case an alert was generated.

Upon completion of this scheme the next step was to introduce care workers
and clients in the project. The ambition was set to generate the participation of 25
clients in the projects which were then followed for a period of 6 months. After
this period all data gathered by the system would be analyzed. Participants were
selected by care workers and asked for their willingness to cooperate. No specific
medical condition was required. On approval the technology was installed in the
house.

The protocol used was evaluated and approved by a local ethical board. The
results of this pilot demonstrated that the technology could be successfully applied
in The Netherlands [5].

The data flow was managed in an efficient way even though there were different
organizations involved. During the pilot period several alerts were generated. Care
workers active in a typical homecare environment regarded positive to the follow
up of these events. In the residential care, however, reactions were less positive;

care workers active in this field found it very hard to identify the additional value of using this infrastructure. Their main argumentation is that they already have regular (and mostly daily) contact with their clients and consequently they are well aware of the condition of the client. From an organizational point the pilot was considered as a success that stimulated all parties to continue.

2.3 *Large Scale Implementation Project*

A new project has been designed and funding could be organized as well. This time through a grant of the ministry of health: the so called "transition program". The project runs from September 2008 to December 2010. The aims of this project are formulated as follows:

- Scale the users of the technology to 200 clients,
- Perform an effect study in the populations of frail elderly and demented persons living at home,
- Define the conditions under which care workers actually use the information derived from activity monitoring. Define the conditions under which this information infrastructure can be regularly used in homecare.

In general terms, the project could use the same infrastructure as was organized during the pilot period. Due to the fact that a specific research protocol had to be designed for the effect study, the application for approval by the ethical board had to be renewed. To set up a group of 25 frail elderly and 25 persons with dementia proved to be a time consuming process. This was especially caused by the fact that the diagnosis on dementia had to be set according to regular care provision standards, instead of by scientific scales. To select these clients, care workers were introduced in the use of the technology system and they were instructed on how to select participants. Both for the effect study and for the monitoring of all events, it was felt important to have a well defined data management system. One of the desired features was that care workers would be able to introduce new data while on the job. Another desired feature was easy communication with other care providers. Setting up such conditions required, would require data introduction using a personal digital assistant PDA. At the start of the new project one of the partners involved created the "Health Care Information System" called HCIS [6]. It contained patient data, history of alerts and the follow up of events using the sequence of trigger (what initiated the alert?), action (what action has been performed?) and outcome (what was the result of the action?). Most of the items were pre-structured. Also some free text items were added. The use of the HCIS required an intensive introduction course which also was prepared as part of the project.

To obtain the required number of participants, the selection process was started by involving the care workers of two regionally operating teams. They were introduced in the use of technology. During regular meetings the results were

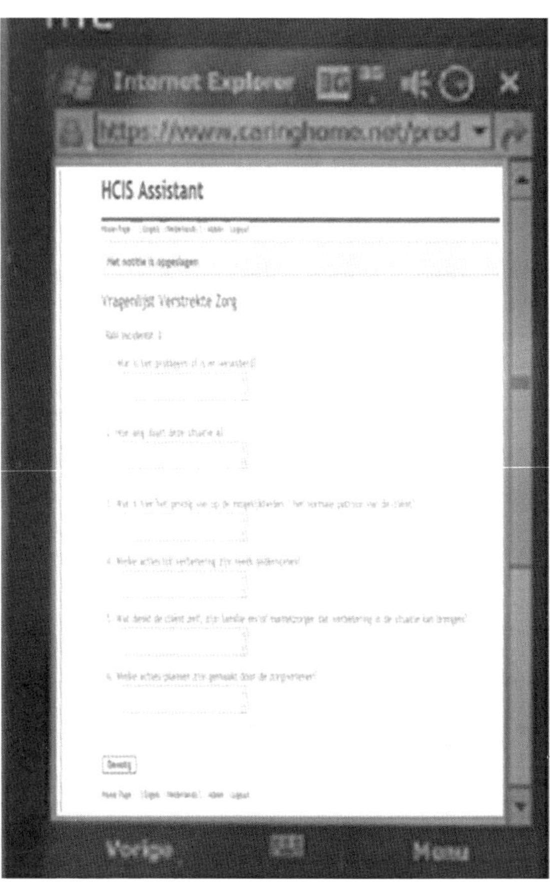

Fig. 3 Questions introduced in the HCIS required to assess the situation that caused an alert

discussed. This was intended to give both the care-workers and the project team feedback on the events. From these meetings it was concluded that the HCIS should not only obtain the operational data, but also an instrument that enabled care workers to describe the rational of their operations. This meant that also the considerations which he or she had during the assessment of the situation prior to the initiation of the action should be included in the HCIS. This was supported by the addition of a set of questions in the HCIS as depicted in Fig. 3.

2.4 On Triggers and Actions

The standard set of the technology uses five infrared motion sensors, a temperature sensor and a communication module. Using this infrastructure the following items can be recorded: bedroom exit, potential bathroom fall, medication events, total activity, nighttime activity, meal preparation, night bathroom activity. By adding

Table 1 Alerts generated from January to July 2010

	J	F	M	A	M	J	J	total
Bedroom exit during night	4	6	8	4	7	7	7	**43**
Overnight bathroom visit	3	0	3	1	2	3	3	**15**
Possible bathroom fall	1	4	5	9	4	5	11	**39**
Meals	0	1	1	0	0	0	0	**2**
Room temperature	0	4	0	1	0	0	30	**35**
(Reduced) activity	3	2	1	3	1	2	5	**17**
Base station dialing in	15	14	16	16	30	20	23	**134**
Connected clients	45	55	64	65	68	75	81	

one or more sensors also wandering behavior can be detected. The system is used in such a way that it can establish an activity pattern that is specific for the person involved. After this learning period, in our case set on 2 weeks, alerts can be generated. Yellow alerts are generated by gradual changes that are supposed to have a limited impact but can become dangerous when the situation persists for longer periods. For instance a reduced number of medication or meal preparation events. Red alerts are given when immediate action is required, for instance when a potential bathroom fall is detected. If client's conditions change because of prolonged absence (for example during vacation), the system can be put on hold by the care provider. In the care protocol all required actions are documented. Table 1 presents the number of red alerts in the period of January 2010 until July 2010. As can be seen from this table the total number of alerts is relatively low.

The fact that several people are involved in the care for each individual and that there is a clear distinction in the follow up measurements between the red and yellow alerts, caused the introduction of quality control measurements. Monthly meetings between care workers in which the events are discussed served this control.

The actions initiated by the alerts involved are of a diverse nature. Initially contact with the client is sought by telephone. This may be followed by a contact to a known informal caregiver living nearby and/or a home-visit to the client. In terms of outcome, the results obtained so far can be described as: reassuring the client, reestablishing their home situation, delivery of first aid and hospitalization.

2.5 Designing a Societal Business Case

Within the framework of the transition program the model in Fig. 4 is used to determine the societal business case [7]. It is essential to note that all future activities described in this activity have to be formulated from the clients perspective. This is done to ascertain that the resulting data will be applicable in the near future. Then, it will be possible to obtain a positive exploitation of this service, even though the environment in which this service will be delivered will

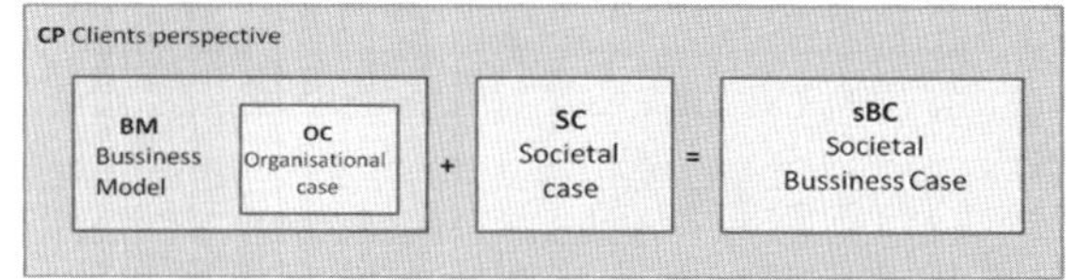

Fig. 4 Model for the development of societal business case

change drastically over time. All services involved must create additional value as seen from the clients' perspective. In the business model section these services are described in detail. In this case it is described what are the target groups of the service (people living independently in need of some care support) to whom this service is delivered (the client themselves and or the informal or formal care provider). It is also described what's the distribution channel of the service to potential clients (internet, personal contact) and what kind of skills and organizational arrangements are required to organize these services. In the organizational paragraph a detailed description and calculation is given on the costs involved in the production of these services. Also the revenues obtained during present operations are given. The results are presented for several years (up to 2014) with a perspective on the development of the service. Next the societal case is described. In this paragraph not only the different stakeholders are described. Also their potential revenues in the application of these services are identified. Calculations are made to see whether a positive exploitation can be obtained. Taken together the result of this exercise gives information on the potential of this innovative approach. In our case the following societal benefits were identified and calculated. These are: (a) a postponement of the admission of these clients to intramural care institution with an average duration of 3 month, (b) a reduced use of societal support (c) less medicine consumption by informal care providers (d) less visits to be delivered by a general practitioner.

It will be clear that this approach gives only a snap-shot of the situation. A lot of yet unforeseeable factors may influence the results. Nevertheless, it appears to become a powerful instrument to organize the discussion between the different stakeholders involved.

The net result of the exercise performed so far by making these kinds of calculations is not the result that under certain assumptions a positive exploitation may be achieved (although that's the result we obtained up to now). The important result is that the healthcare insurance board and several other care organizations active in the region are considering to participate in the project. Furthermore, conditions are created to organize a measurement of the effects using a control group as well.

3 Outcome of the Project

The result of the project obtained so far can be described as follows:

- More than 120 clients have participated in the project with an average duration of 214 ± 168 days up to now with a total of 53 person years,

- More than 44 care providers are introduced in the project and have active knowledge of aim, principles and results at the client level,
- Three different care organizations are supporting some of their clients with technology.
- A regional information infrastructure has been organized,
- At the client level, several examples of positive action of the system are gathered,
- A training program has been organized and evaluated to get care workers acquainted with the use of technology as part of care provision,
- Informal carers are supported with information that is relevant to their care provision task,
- The project has been identified as an innovative approach to make care support sustainable.

Viewed from the perspective of the care organization the following outcome has been achieved as well; the use of this technology contributes to what can be described as a social innovation. The presence of the technology in the social network of a person stimulates that network (of potential informal carers) to operate more efficiently in monitoring wellbeing of the elderly person. Up to now this task was delegated more or less to the homecare organization. In essence, a homecare organization is not adequately well equipped to take this responsibility. Thus, in an early stage of the disease process, fundamental changes in the living situation have to be introduced, most likely leading towards intramural uptake of the client. To the person with a developing process of dementia living independently, the support of the social network may contribute to the continuation of the situation of independent living safely for a prolonged period.

4 Internal Influences on Development and Outcome

First of all the organization involved in the project needs to have a strong and persisting commitment to the activity. The introduction of activity monitoring is an innovative process with a high risk; the commitment of (the management of) the organization is a prerequisite. In the initial pilot project it was essential that participating care workers have an open mind to the general usage of technology in care. This is due to the fact that all members of the project team involved are unfamiliar with the possible effects of the application of this technology. Based on the results of the pilot a transition to regular practice was made. Care workers participating in the project were members of three out of 40 of the care providers's care teams. These teams incorporated the application into their regular practice as much as possible. An introduction program, taking into account the experiences of the pilot, was given to these care workers about the usage of the technology. During the project it became evident that an increasing group of care workers had to become involved. This introduced the need to influence their attitude towards the application of technology in care.

Care receivers are also important partners in the development. In this specific case it is positive that the burden to initiate in the project is low; their activities remain unchanged and are not interfered by the project. Also the fact that an abstract interpretation of their activities is made (indicated by a traffic light mechanism), instead of a direct view of the activities reduces the potential burden.

During the course of the project it became evident that organizational and financial conditions for the provision of homecare would change in the nearby future. Thus it became apparent that insight in the cost structure would be necessary to the project as well, resulting in the development of a societal business case.

5 External Influences on Development and Outcome

The project started with the ambition to set up a way of service delivery while recognizing the prospect of increased demand of care and a reduction of labour force. This prospect is initiated merely by demographic changes. The care organization has invested a limited amount of own funding in the project. In co-operation with HSZuyd, additional sources were sought. The developmental process was communicated to organizations in public health services (like the regional health insurance board) to initiate and safe-guard future financing schemes.

The care organization as initiator of the project remained active in organizing new ways of care delivery. During this project they also initiated activities in other domains. They were also able to broaden the use of technology in care in greater parts of their organization. The consortium contained more care organizations. Although these remained active in the project, they were not able to develop a positive attitude towards the use of technology in care and consequently they did not initiate accompanying activities. They remained reactive instead of becoming innovative.

Within the project, no legal issues were prominent except the issue of an ethical evaluation. Compared to other projects in which technology is involved, the ethical issues are of minor importance. Two factors are important; there is no interference with activity performance itself and the data management is done anonymously.

Right at the start of the project it became clear that the care organization by itself will not be able to set all the conditions required to create a workable solution. The scale of operation to fully support this service in its own hands will not be reached. For example, the organization is not able to maintain a 24/7 call center. Thus a co-operation with others will be necessary. In this project an effective co-operation with the regional ambulance care service center was introduced to serve as a 24/7 call center. The care organization is active as a care organization currently active as part of Dutch healthcare service that is regulated by the AWBZ-act [8]. The Dutch government has initiated a process under which this legislation changed. The role of local organizations, like municipalities, is becoming more and more important with regard to the financial arrangements. End users will also become a financial actor; they will have to pay in a direct way for the service given to them. These gradual changes introduce insecurity on how future exploitation of this new service will become possible. As a consequence of these developments a societal business case had to be developed during the project.

The insecure situation with regard of the long term structure of healthcare also had its effects on the project partners and its consortium. Right at the start of the project two care provider organizations had to withdraw from the project. At that time they were not able to deliver the effort needed. This resulted in a much slower entry of clients into the project. To the consortium this introduced the need to identify new partners. This caused a continued inventory in the regional network of care organizations. In the course of the project this rendered success as two new organizations were able to enter and supported several clients with this kind of service.

The project is directed towards the assembly and interpretation of activities performed by a person in their own home environment. The processes of data gathering and interpretation may interfere with the persons privacy. To assess the ethical dilemmas involved herein, the protocol for this evaluation was evaluated and approved by a local ethical board. As a result, strict information rules were to be maintained. This also limited the possibility to incorporate participants with dementia in the early stages of disease developments into the research group. Only clients diagnosed according to the criteria of present healthcare practice could be included; meaning that the dementia status was prominently available. As a consequence of this situation the informal carers of the participants also became a relevant group to this project and they were included in the data gathering as well.

6 User Aspects

The introduction of new care workers as participants in the project, regardless whether they are a member of the care organization, caused the need for an introductory or educational program. This program was developed as part of the project and will also serve as a demonstrative approach to future applications of care at a distance. Also an introductory course will be developed aimed at informal carers. This will enable them to get familiar with the use of the information generated by the infrastructure.

As part of both the pilot and the large scale implementation project, the user related aspects were covered as well. At the client and at the informal carer's level, interviews were kept at regular intervals. These are directed towards the effects noted by them. At the end of the pilot period, in which 24 clients were involved, only one client indicates to be unsatisfied with the system. Most of the clients are satisfied by the possibility that the information (gathered based upon their activities) can be shared with their relatives. Half of the users is willing to recommend the use of this system to colleagues and friends. During the pilot, care workers were less positive about the technology than the clients. Nevertheless, they acknowledged to receive information on the clients' functioning which they could not have obtained otherwise. They were a bit disturbed by the frequent baseline alerts and were not yet able to interpret them. During the pilot they experienced the handling of the information obtained in this way as an extra effort. During the follow-up investigation the introduction of the HCIS gave them an insight in the use of information that could be directly related to their professional functioning, thereby improving the net result of the application. Data gathering of information on aspects of use during the large scale implementation project is still ongoing.

7 General Aspects

This project is an ongoing but promising investigation. Conclusions of care givers in the area of quality of life, as can be noted from their reactions during interviews, remain positive. Care workers are satisfied with their increased insight in actual behavior of their clients living in their own homes; it is unprecedented that they have this kind of information.

Information on the potential of activity monitoring was spread through contacts with care workers of the care organization through regular contacts. Also potential clients were informed. Information leaflets and a website (www.veranderingzien.nl) were made to communicate to care workers and the general public. During the project care organization in the region were kept informed about the development of the project. To two of them this lead to interest to participate with some of their clients as well.

8 Conclusion

At this stage of the developments it has become clear that activity monitoring is an application that may support individual clients in their safety and supports them in the continuation of independent living. Care workers are becoming more and more interested to work with this kind of technology; to some of them the project has given insight and understanding of the potential of technology and may have to support their work as a nurse in a direct way. The project has opened the perspective to support teamwork in everyday practice by using information and communication tools like the HCIS as an efficient alternative to oral communication.

References

1. Barberger-Gateau P, Fabrigoule C, Helmer C, Rouch I, Dartigues JF. Functional impairment in instrumental activities of daily living: an early clinical sign of dementia? J Am Geriatr Soc. 1999; 47(4):456–62.
2. Gure TR, Kabeto MU, Plassman BL, Piette JD, Langa KM. Series A; Biological Sciences and Medical Sciences. Differences in functional impairment across subtypes of dementia. J Gerontol. 2010; 65(4):434–41. Epub 2009 Dec 17.

3. Martin S, Kelly G, Kernohan WG, McCreight B, Nugent C. Smart home technologies for health and social care support. Cochrane Database System, Rev. 2008 Oct 8;(4): CD006412.
4. Glascock A, Kutzik D editors. Handbook of research on IT and clinical data administration in healthcare. A care informatics approach to telehomecare applications. IGI Publishing, Hershey, PA; 2009. pp. 368–382.
5. Willems ChG, Glascock AP, Kutzik DM, Rietman J. The role of an informatics-based telehome care in a person-centered service delivery model: findings from a feasibility study in the Netherlands. Report HsZuyd 2010.
6. Glascock AP, Kutzik D. Embrace the chaos, it's not noise: Lessons learned from non-traditional environments. Int J Mobile Hum Comput Interact. 2009;1:22–36.
7. www.tplz.nl visited July 29th 2010.
8. Department of welfare health and sports. Healthcare in the Netherlands; home care. The Hague, The Netherlands, 2005; 76–80. Downloaded July 29th 2010 from http://english. minvws.nl/en/folders/cz/2005/primary-health-care.asp.

A Retrospective View of a Rehabilitation Homecare Scenario for Cardiac Patients

Oliver Koslowski, Myriam Lipprandt, Clemens Busch, Marco Eichelberg, Frerk Müller, Detlev Willemsen, Gökçe Banu Laleci Ertürkmen, Asuman Dogac and Andreas Hein

Abstract The SAPHIRE project aimed to develop an intelligent healthcare monitoring and decision support system on a platform integrating the wireless medical sensor data with hospital information systems. In this paper one of the two demonstrator environments—the homecare scenario—is described from the medical and technical point of view. A retrospective view of the technical and medical internal challenges of the homecare scenario of the project is given. Also

O. Koslowski (✉)
ATLAS Elektronik, Bremen, Germany
e-mail: oliver.koslowski@atlas-elektronik.com

M. Lipprandt · M. Eichelberg · F. Müller · A. Hein
OFFIS—Institute for Information Technology, Oldenburg, Germany
e-mail: myriam.lipprandt@offis.de

M. Eichelberg
e-mail: marco.eichelberg@offis.de

F. Müller
e-mail: frerk.mueller@offis.de

A. Hein
e-mail: andreas.hein@offis.de

C. Busch · D. Willemsen
Schüchtermann-Schiller'sche Kliniken, Bad Rothenfelde, Germany
e-mail: cbusch@schuechtermann-klinik.de

D. Willemsen
e-mail: dwillemsen@schuechtermann-klinik.de

G. B. L. Ertürkmen · A. Dogac
Software Research, Development and Consultation Ltd, Ankara, Turkey
e-mail: gokce@srdc.com.tr

A. Dogac
e-mail: asuman@srdc.com.tr

Commun Med Care Compunetics (2011) 3: 181–196
DOI: 10.1007/8754_2011_20
© Springer-Verlag Berlin Heidelberg 2011
Published Online: 8 May 2011

the external challenges that influenced the project, like economic aspects and legal issues, are being discussed. Furthermore, an outlook on the follow-up project OSAmI is given with regards to the experience learned from SAPHIRE (http://www.srdc.com.tr/metu-srdc/webpage/projects/saphire).

Keywords Homecare · Tele-rehabilitation · Cardiologic rehabilitation systems

1 The SAPHIRE Project

SAPHIRE (Intelligent Healthcare Monitoring based on Semantic Interoperability Platform) was a project funded by the European Commission as part of the 6th Framework Programme. The project had a contract period of 2.5 years, from the 01.01.2006 to 30.06.2008 and the total cost of the project amounted to 2.9 MEUR. SAPHIRE was built upon the results of an earlier European Commission funded project, IST-1-002103 Artemis [1], which developed a semantic web service-based P2P infrastructure for the interoperability of medical information systems. The Artemis system enables healthcare institutes to exchange electronic healthcare records in an interoperable manner through semantically enriched web services and semantic mediation. As the subtitle of the project suggests, the aim of SAPHIRE [2, 3] was the development of a system that uses a platform for semantic interoperability in order to provide services for an intelligent monitoring of patient data. The overall SAPHIRE vision is presented in Fig. 1.

Patient monitoring at home or at a hospital was achieved by a set of mobile and wireless connected sensors assigned to a single patient. Agent technology was used to collect and combine or fuse sensor data. The "agent behaviour" was supported by intelligent decision support systems based on clinical practice guidelines (CDSS). The patient histories stored in medical information systems were accessed through semantically enriched Web services and medical standards (like CDA or XDS [4, 5]) to tackle the interoperability problem. In this way, not only the observations received as patient's physiological signs data during a conventional diagnostic process but also the patient medical history (such as previous diagnoses, medication list, allergies and adverse drug reactions), clinical guidelines [6], physiological signs received (continuously) from wireless medical sensors and the patient care plan all affected the clinical path to be followed. Due to the complexity of clinical standards and practice guidelines, healthcare professionals have difficulties in understanding and applying these guidelines in the clinical care setting. This necessitates computerized decision support systems automating clinical guidelines to support the health professionals. One of the major challenges in developing computerized decision support systems was accessing the many disparate data sources needed to retrieve patient-specific information. This led to a distributed architecture with an information infrastructure that requires safeguards to maintain security and privacy of patient data. Patient identification and medical

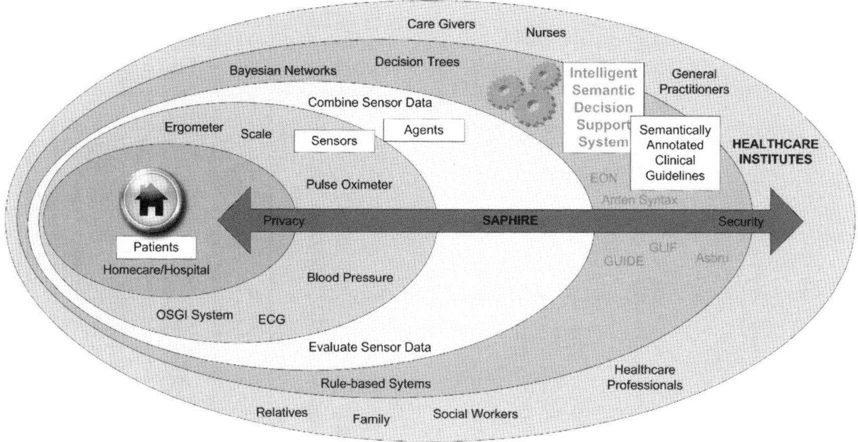

Fig. 1 Conceptual overview of the SAPHIRE project

records cannot be disclosed indiscriminately and different healthcare providers have different access rights. The SAPHIRE project proposed comprehensive security and privacy mechanisms to complement the infrastructure. While providing these confidentiality and privacy mechanisms, the EU directives 95/46/EC [7] and 2002/58/EC [8] presenting the general principles of processing of personal data, and in particular Recommendation R(97)5 of the Council of Europe discussing protection of medical data collected and processed automatically were taken into account.

To show the feasibility of the SAPHIRE framework, two pilot applications were developed. One of these pilot applications was deployed in a hospital environment as an intelligent clinical decision support system guiding the healthcare professionals for patient care based on data gathered from sensors, and medical information systems. The second pilot application was a homecare application, where the patient's medical status was monitored remotely through sensors. Based on the infrastructure provided by the SAPHIRE project, the healthcare institutes deployed intelligent decision support systems for implementing appropriate clinical guidelines.

The homecare pilot application was deployed and tested in Lower Saxony in Germany, where Schüchtermann-Schiller'sche Kliniken (SSK) is located. The goal of this pilot application was to continuously register the relevant data that could indicate an endangerment to the patient and to automatically transmit the data in digital form from the patient's home to the supervising institute, i.e. SSK's Rehabilitation Centre Bad Rothenfelde. At the same time, an intelligent and automated processing and evaluation of data was needed at the supervising centre, providing an alarm as soon as a patient left a pre-defined "corridor". This review focuses on the homecare scenario of the SAPHIRE project.

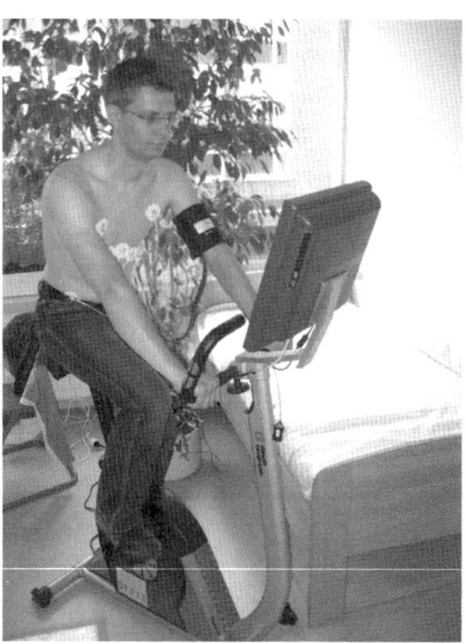

Fig. 2 Patient during the exercise training at home

1.1 The SAPHIRE Homecare Scenario

The homecare scenario targeted patients in their phase III rehabilitation. Whereas the hospital scenario dealt with patients in the sub-acute phase in the hospital, the homecare scenario aimed toward patients after successful treatment and phase I/II rehabilitation. The goal of the homecare scenario was to facilitate a safe, medically supervised training at the patient's home. The rationale behind this scenario had several aims. Physical exercise training is, together with appropriate medication, the most important factor to influence risk factors in a positive way. It can decrease blood pressure and blood lipids as well as increase glucose metabolism. It can lead to a reduction of re-hospitalization through a prolonged, supervised secondary prevention.

The core element of the system was a bicycle ergometer (see Fig. 2). A 15" panel PC had been attached to the ergometer replacing the original control unit. The core sensor for the system was a twelve lead ECG. Alongside with the ECG, the patient received a pulse oximeter and a blood pressure sensor.

The panel PC with its touch screen not only served as user interface for the patient, but also as a gateway that gathered the data from the sensors, controlled the ergometer load and connected the patient's home with the rehabilitation clinic. In this way training plans could be updated and training sessions could be monitored remotely (see Fig. 3).

1.2 Motivation for Homecare Cardiologic Rehabilitation Systems

Cardiovascular diseases (CVD) are the leading cause of death in the world [9], and cause nearly half of all deaths in Europe (48%) and in the EU (42%) [10]. Due to

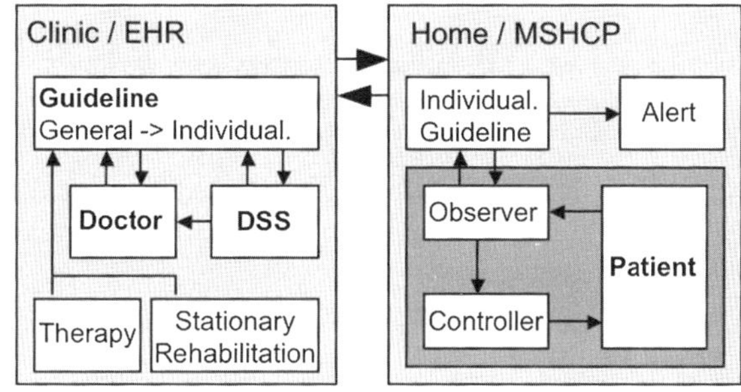

Fig. 3 Information flow between clinic (individualization of training guideline) and the patient's home (alarm system and trainings controller) [3]

demographic change ("ageing society"), the prevalence of CVD is expected to increase in the future, which means that they will be one of the major burdens of diseases that need to be addressed with sustainable prevention programs. The treatment of people with chronic diseases over their lifetime costs 3.5 times more than the treatment of others, and accounts for 80% of all hospital bed days and 96% of home care visits [11]. One important factor for the health outcome of CVD patients after an acute event or cardiac surgery is cardiac rehabilitation. According to the European Association for Cardiovascular Prevention and Rehabilitation (EACPR), ambulatory (outpatient) rehabilitation programs are needed in order to achieve the comprehensive goals of cardiac rehabilitation and maintain them over time [12]. One key aspect of such ambulatory rehabilitation is exercise training, which can reduce further deterioration of the disease and prevent expensive readmission. For high-risk CVD patients, however, supervision and monitoring by health professionals are required.

Patients in Germany with severe CVD currently receive an in-patient rehabilitation program of 3–5 weeks after acute treatment. During this time the health status required for a reintegration of the patient should be achieved. Therefore, the restoration of the patient's physical capabilities through an exercise adapted to the patient's individual condition is in focus of the rehabilitation treatment. Furthermore, patients receive training and consultancy with regard to reducing the avoidable risk factors.

However, after a cardiac event, lifelong secondary prevention is crucial to avert further progress of the disease, maintain at least the current health status and improve the cardiac prognosis. Currently only 50% of all patients participate in a phase II rehabilitation in Europe, according to the Euroaspire study [13]. The American Heart Association (AHA) as well as the European Association of Cardiovascular Prevention and Rehabilitation (EACPR) define core components for a lifelong secondary prevention of cardiac heart disease. The prevention aims to enhance the modifiable cardiac risk factors, which are weight management, nutritional counselling, blood pressure management, lipid management, smoking cessation and physical activity counselling [14, 15].

After a cardiac event and the following phase II rehabilitation, cardiac risk factors are well adjusted. However, a study has shown that 1 year after discharge the risk factors are comparable to the time before the cardiac event and in some cases even deteriorate [16]. These data are elevated from patients participating to phase II rehabilitation. It can be assumed that for the 50% of all patients not taking part in any rehabilitation, the risk factors will deteriorate in the same manner or even worse.

Regular physical activity and exercise training have a positive influence on risk factors like hypertension, diabetes, obesity and dyslipidemia, which are not sufficiently treated already 6 month after a cardiac event as shown before. The American College of Sports Medicine, the American Heart Association, the European Society of Cardiology and the German Society of Rehabilitation and Prevention recommend a minimal amount of physical exercise for at least five times a week for 30 min in moderate intensity [15]. However, those guidelines only suggest physical endurance exercise in general. Several studies have shown that an individualized exercise regime will even increase the effect of physical activity. A controlled training that has been adjusted to individual needs can optimize the secondary prevention. An ideal way for controlled training is a bicycle ergometer. Exact power and time can be adjusted and different physical parameters like heart frequency, ECG, oxygen saturation, and blood pressure can be monitored easily. For patients with high risk factors, monitored exercise is strongly recommended and is an integral part of phase II rehabilitation.

Typically an exercise session on a bicycle ergometer is divided in three or five phases. It starts with a warm-up phase, which is normally preset on an individual low intensity (approximately 30–40% of the individual maximal performance). The amount of time depends on the total time of the exercise session (e.g. 3 mins within a total time of 30 min). During the second part the intensity is increased to its training load in a linear way (within a 30 min exercise unit it would take 2 min to raise the exercise load). The third part is the actual training. It lasts at least 20 min and it is adjusted to the individual need. The forth and fifth section are congruent to the warm-up and the developing phase in time and load but vice versa. Very weak patients would exercise with so-called interval training. It is divided in three phases (warm-up, training and cool-down). The training is characterized with alternation of low intensity and high intensity loads, typically divided in two to one intervals, meaning for example 40 s on low intensity and 20 s on high intensity load, plus three to 5 min of continuous low load as warm-up and cool-down phase.

Today, many heart centres offer so-called "cardiac sports groups" where patients can train regularly under professional supervision as a means of secondary prevention. While in urban areas a sufficient number of cardiac sports groups are offered, only a small number of such groups are offered in rural regions, requiring participants to accept significant journeys. In this context the introduction of tele-medical supervision systems for exercise training at home seems reasonable.

2 Internal Challenges on the Homecare Cardiologic Rehabilitation System

2.1 Technical Challenges and Results

From a technical point of view the project allowed for the construction and testing of a platform for wireless medical sensors. One of the concerns at the beginning of the project had been the bandwidth required for sensor data. Calculations based on the theoretical bandwidth of bluetooth connections and the required data rate for a typical 12-lead ECG suggested that bandwidth would be no issue. While this was shown to be true, bluetooth connectivity still proved to be problematic. During numerous sessions a sensor would simply not connect to the sensor gateway and the reasons remained and still remain unknown. While wireless sensors can greatly increase a patient's mobility in the hospital scenario, that feature is not really necessary in the homecare scenario where the sensors are most likely to be used in conjunction with the ergometer bike as the sensor gateway. This is why follow-up projects re-implemented a similar sensor setup without wireless connections in order to reduce the cost of the systems and to increase the reliability.

The handling of sensors (especially the placement of the ECG electrodes at the chest) requires support. Contrary to the situation at a clinic no support is possible by the medical staff. Consequently, the exercise plan was complemented with visual instructions on how to place the sensors (see Fig. 4) and if possible by automatic tests (e.g. consistency measurements) to determine the proper functionality of the sensors.

The project proposal did not suggest a specific method for alert generation. In the project a rule-based approach was used since it was the best approximation of the devices already in use, and because rule engines like Jess were known to be fast enough for the task at hand. In [17] we discussed the performance of this rule-based system. While its sensitivity was generally satisfactory, its specificity was too low to allow for training sessions without interruptions. A rule-based system can only be as good as the data it is evaluating, and in the case of a training scenario, motion artefacts make sensor data unreliable. Figure 5 shows a typical ECG signal of a patient in motion. The signal is so noisy that automatic interpretation proved to be well beyond the capabilities of the third-party software used in the project. Even though no major adverse cardiac events (MACE) were encountered during the trial sessions with patients of the Schüchtermann-Klinik, the software reported a whole plethora of serious events that triggered alerts. A simple rule-based approach works fine in situations where sensor data is not riddled with motion artefacts, as shown in the hospital scenario of the project.

While the overall technical results were satisfactory for a demonstrator that was designed as a proof-of-concept, they demanded further research to increase the robustness of the signal interpretation.

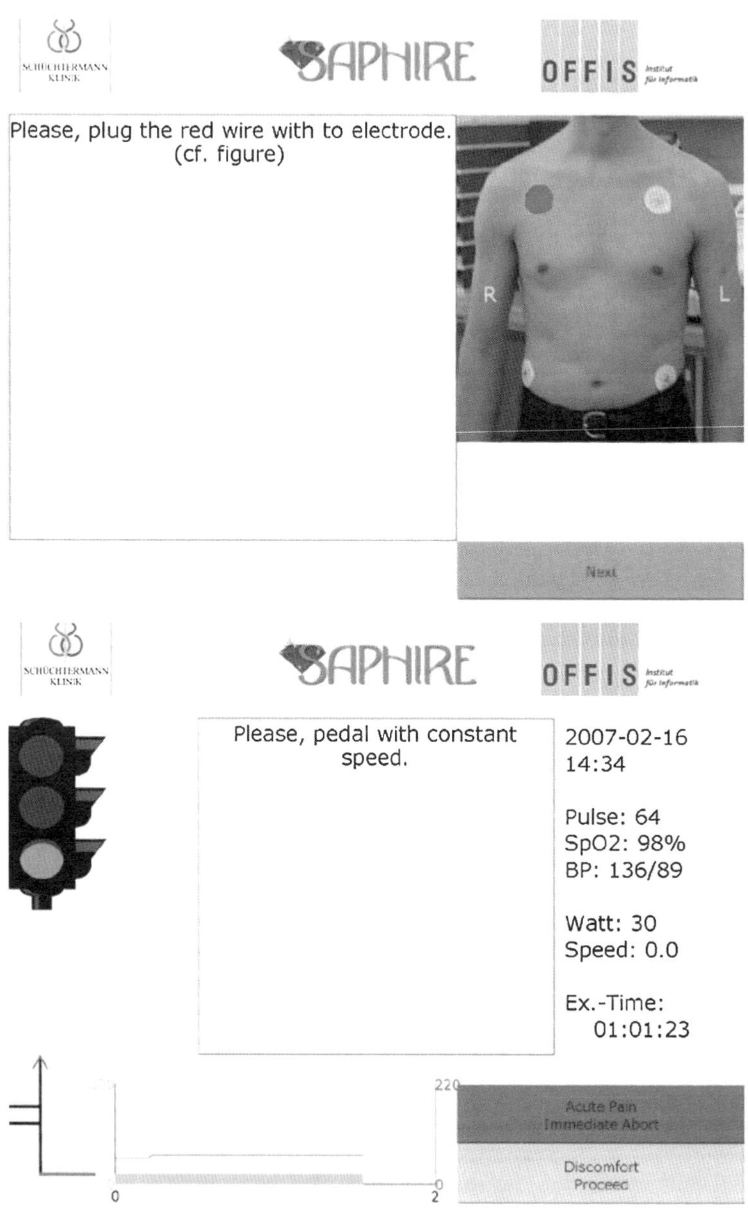

Fig. 4 Screenshots from the touch screen: status of the placement of the ECG electrodes (*left*) and state of the training with traffic lights and current/desired load and speed

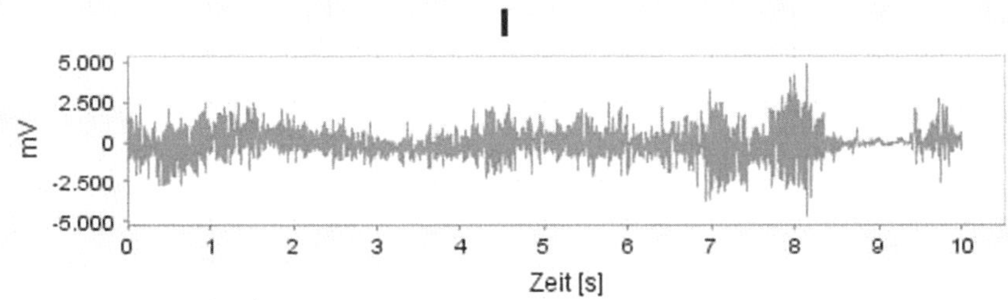

Fig. 5 ECG of Einthoven (lead I) with severe motion artefacts

2.2 Medical Challenges and Results

The project succeeded in terms of proof of concept. A functional system could be realised allowing online supervision of ECG, blood pressure and oxygen saturation. Furthermore the training system itself was able to supervise an individual exercise according to the "agent" based standard defined. Those standards had been derived from current guidelines of electro-physical definitions (e.g. tachycardia, couplets, triplets, etc.), blood pressure recommendations and oxygen saturation for exercise training.

However, some requirements could not be realised in the final demonstrator. Even though a full 12-lead ECG was recorded and transmitted online, only one lead could be displayed by the GUI. The system crashed easily in case someone did not choose the "right" way of the workflow. Furthermore, it had been intended to interact remotely with the system in the patients' home, but this could not be realised. These minor failures could have been solved with a prolonged and product-oriented project. However, within this research project the main aim was the proof of concept. Yet based on experiences made and apart from these technical inaccuracies some conceptual additions could be identified to be crucial for further exploitation:

1. *Flexibility in regard to patient needs*: In the current project the patient had to put on all sensors, even if some sensors would not have been necessarily important. For example, a young CHD patient with a good lung function, after a minor infarct would not need oxygen saturation or blood pressure measurement in everyday exercise training. But the SAPHIRE system could not easily be adapted to such a scenario.
2. *Everyday usability*: Unfortunately, this could only be tested by a stable day-to-day routine usage over a prolonged time for at least three to 6 month. It is very likely that a 12-lead ECG with electrodes that need to be attached to the skin on precisely defined locations on the patient's body is not reasonable for use in day-to-day practice.
3. *Online supervision of training*: This feature requires a broadband connection at both sides, and furthermore supervisor and patient need to commonly arrange certain dates for a supervised training e.g. by telephone.

However, in order to develop a more flexible system in the successor project OSAmI, a much more flexible concept has been developed. Usability aspects have been integrated from the very beginning developing the demonstrator in a three-cycle loop. In this way an early integration of the end-users could be realised. The concept of the OSAmI system distinguishes three levels of training settings depending on the individual health status of the patient and on individual demands. Firstly, a patient can receive face-to-face online training with integrated audio–video conferencing as well as online remote adaptable training time load and thresholds. Secondly, a patient can join a "group training". He/she logs on at a certain time into the hospital network and simultaneously exercises as part of a group of people. A supervisor monitors the remote training sessions. In both cases a standard broadband connection would be necessary. Thirdly, the patient is allowed to train at any time. A predefined training will lead through the session. In case of any threshold violation the system stops immediately. A report is generated in all cases of online and offline training. The last scenario allows stable patient to exercise on their own whenever they feel like. Once a day the ergometer goes online and sends its reports and queries for updates. In case something changed surprisingly or a serious alarm is detected, the report is sent immediately and the supervisor is informed.

3 Medical and Patient Centric User Aspects

Acceptability, usefulness and usability have been part of the evaluation of the project. Generally two aspects had to be evaluated. On the one hand the supervision/monitoring software with an integrated administrative part as well as the setting of individual training sessions, and the online monitoring part. On the other side, it was necessary to evaluate the end-user/patient software with the integrated sensors. For that reason the opinion of patients and supervisors was of great interest. A questionnaire was developed to measure the first reactions and feelings towards the system. Different aspects of usability were asked. Unfortunately the system was not stable enough to monitor patients for a longer period and to use it in day-to-day practice. However, supervisors were convinced of the potential of the software and could not identify any major disadvantages [18].

The patient-side was tested after several training sessions. It was our interest to see how a user would get used to the operation of the training software and to the application of the sensors. The results were also quite promising, which means that the system could in the future play an important role for secondary prevention for cardiac patients [18].

The main concern of the end users as well as the supervisors was the safety and reliability of the system. However, as already mentioned, SAPHIRE was a research project. Therefore, the intensive testing, improvement and re-testing cycles needed to achieve a stable system could not be realized during the time-frame of the project.

4 External Challenges on the Homecare Cardiologic Rehabilitation System

4.1 Economic Aspects

Aside from the aspect of the patient's quality of life, economic aspects played a role in the motivation for and the development of the project. The same aspects influence the commercial exploitation of the project results. Very few research projects can be exploited directly, but still the exploitation of the project results for SAPHIRE proved to be more difficult than initially expected. SAPHIRE as a product would have to "survive" in an economic niche that is not defined by an open market but a system that depends on the cooperation of several partners. A patient is not the intended (direct) customer of a product derived from the SAPHIRE system. Without technical and medical support, a patient would gain little from the product. Furthermore, it seems unlikely that many patients would be willing to pay the full price for the equipment, so some reimbursement by the health insurance would be necessary. However, currently health insurance companies are reluctant to pay for products for secondary prevention, especially if the long-term effects have not been fully proven yet. The beneficial effects as well as the economic feasibility need to be proven in clinical trials. This was out of the scope of the SAPHIRE project. In order to be useful, the business model would also require the assistance from rehabilitation clinics. The coordination of these partners can be difficult and proved to be a too daunting task at the end of SAPHIRE, which is why further follow-up research projects were acquired.

4.2 Legal Issues

Since both scenarios were tested with patients, these small-scale trials had to be approved by the respective ethics committees. Furthermore, informed consent by the patients involved in the trials was necessary. However, the exploitation of the project results requires additional measures because of the European Medical Device Directive. The most pertinent question was the degree of certification required by the directive. Whereas it seemed certain that the hardware had to be certified, the question of how to deal with the software parts was not fully answered during the course of the project.

The Medical Device Directive (MDD) 93/42/EEC and its update through directive 2007/47/EC define a set of requirements regarding the safety and quality of medical devices. The original MDD from 1993, which was subsequently transformed into national laws in Europe, defines medical devices as follows: "*Medical device* means any instrument, apparatus, appliance, material or other article, whether used alone or in combination, including the software necessary for its proper application intended by the manufacturer to be used for human beings for the purpose of diagnosis, prevention, monitoring, treatment or alleviation of disease, [...]".

The role of software systems in the context of the original MDD was subject to debate and needed to be clarified based on the revision process that eventually lead to directive 2007/47/EC. The paragraph defining medical devices has been updated as follows: "*Medical device* means any instrument, apparatus, appliance, software, material or other article, whether used alone or in combination, together with any accessories, including the software intended by its manufacturer to be used specifically for diagnostic and/or therapeutic purposes and necessary for its proper application, intended by the manufacturer to be used for human beings for the purpose of diagnosis, prevention, monitoring, treatment or alleviation of disease [...]".

Under this definition, not only the hardware components (sensors, computer and ergometer) and the local load controller at the ergometer have to be considered as an active medical device that is regulated by the MDD, but also the CDSS, the communication channel to the clinic and the management and storage of the training reports and the sensor data. The most immediate effect is described in the updated Annex I: "For devices which incorporate software or which are medical software in themselves, the software must be validated according to the state of the art taking into account the principles of development life-cycle, risk management, validation and verification."

The last three aspects—risk management, validation and verification—have been neglected in many CDSS. If a system is sought to go beyond a research project, the requirements of the MDD need to be fulfilled.

5 Dissemination Strategy

In the SAPHIRE project, the dissemination strategy was planned and published in reports [19] that were updated every 6 months. With partners from academia, medicine and industry a wide range of dissemination options was exploited. The dissemination strategy identified the need to address the scientific community, industrial audiences as potential service providers and of course potential users. The Schüchtermann-Klinik as the medical partner in the homecare scenario addressed mostly medical audiences in papers. OFFIS as technical partner tried to address both academic and non-academic audiences.

A 'general' roadmap was designed for dissemination and awareness activities to take place as part of the project activities. The industrial IT supplier partners were asked to adapt this 'generic' roadmap for individual national markets. This was done jointly with the research partners. Specific attention was paid to the dissemination of project's clinical results.

Though not part of the contractual commitments, all SAPHIRE consortium members recognized the need for establishing a SAPHIRE community, which would consist of several different types of actors that are positioned along the

SAPHIRE value chain. These range from 'competing' research or academic institutions to industry actors to potential uptakers and users of the SAPHIRE technology and solutions. The SAPHIRE consortium created a contacts database with individuals and institutions that were contacted and asked if they were interested in receiving a SAPHIRE newsletter. Six newsletters were published during the course of the project and can still be found at [19].

One important cornerstone of the dissemination efforts was the identification of project assets. Some assets, such as the software architecture, are intangible. The dissemination activities greatly benefited from tangible assets such as the hospital scenario demonstrator or the homecare demonstrator. The homecare demonstrator could be transported easily and was shown in several venues and congresses. In order to jump-start dissemination activities, early prototypes for both scenarios were prepared even before some of the sensors were available in their final specifications. Because the demonstrators were tangible, they were suitable for presentations on TV. METU had the opportunity to present the hospital scenario on Turkey's national television and OFFIS was featured on local television. The homecare demonstrator was on display at CeBIT (the biggest IT trade show in the world) and at MEDICA, which is Europe's largest medical trade show.

6 Outlook on OSAmI

In the opinion of the technical partner OFFIS as well as the end-user Schüchter-mann Klinik, the SAPHIRE approach is the right way to offer a wide range of secondary prevention for patients with chronic heart disease. The first results could be brought into the ongoing project OSAmI (Open Source Ambient Intelligence Commons). The technical approach differs strongly from the SAPHIRE project, but the conceptual idea of a supervised online training system for cardiac patients has been expanded in several ways.

In OSAmI the tele-rehabilitation of patients with cardiovascular disease also takes place in the home environment, but additionally an outdoor training is developed. The patient is equipped with a set of medical sensors like an ECG, blood pressure, oxygen saturation and pulse sensor to monitor the heart frequency. In case of ergometer training the sensors are directly linked to the control computer. The sensor data are collected, analysed and fused during a training session to control the ergometer load and to avoid any overload of the patient. Also an alarm system must give feedback about the current health status while exercising. The need of an individualized training plan that is adapted over time makes a connection to a clinic necessary. Also training reports including all vital parameters and medical events like alarms must be transmitted to the clinic after every training session. The training reports represent the patient's health status, history and fitness level. Based on this information, a medical supervisor can review every training report to generate a new, appropriately adapted training plan that can be transmitted back to the home-based rehabilitation system. For interoperability reasons, the gathered vital parameters should be transmitted in a standard format (CDA [4]). In addition to the bicycle ergometer training, a tele-rehabilitation application should support different sport activities that can be performed to increase the physical fitness level, such as nordic walking or jogging. The challenge in the development of such a system is to adapt from the laboratory conditions to the tele-rehabilitation system at home. The characteristics of a clinical setting give complete control and information about the patient's health status during the training phase. This allows for progress monitoring, emergency detection and adaption of exercise level by a medical professional without being face-to-face with the patient all the time. Compared to the SAPHIRE system OSAmI is mature on a conceptual level.

Besides the medical requirements, the objectives of OSAmI are also to enable interoperability, maintainability, and reliability of complex, distributed systems as they are typically used in medical monitoring applications including homecare. The management of medical devices and an automated configuration is also in scope. The goal of the OSAmI platform is to significantly simplify the development of distributed monitoring and assisting systems, thus enabling new forms of delivery of care.

In contrast to SAPHIRE, the OSAmI application is extended with outdoor training and an indoor training in "offline mode". Furthermore, the system architecture is quite different; the service-oriented architecture (SOA) paradigm is consistently used in the OSAmI architecture. The communication between sensors and home care unit (hence gateway) uses Device Profile for Web Services (DPWS) [20] as a standardized up-to-date service protocol. It enables newly attached sensors to be discovered dynamically and is easily supported by common SOA based web-service toolkits [21].

The users' needs and requirements regarding to their impairment or age are also in focus of OSAmI. Classical user interfaces and interface design for mobile devices should be context-aware to reduce the cognitive overload and adapt to the different situations during a training session [22].

The development cycle contains three integration and validation cycles of the demonstrator. In every cycle the domain analysis and architectural changes are characterised to show the evolution of the demonstrator during the project.

7 Conclusion

The aim of the SAPHIRE project to develop a system that uses a platform for semantic interoperability in order to provide services for an intelligent monitoring of patient data was successfully reached. Despite the indisputable results of SAPHIRE, it can be stated that flexibly combinable and co-operating embedded devices and software components are still difficult to implement, especially in the healthcare sector, due to the multitude of specialised, partly proprietary communication protocols and interfaces [23, 24]. The results from SAPHIRE highlighted the fact that in the domain of homecare sensor data are of a lesser quality because of motion artefacts and instable bluetooth connections. An autonomous alarm system is, therefore, very difficult to develop. Also the guidance of patients to deal with professional medical equipment at home (e.g. 12-lead ECG) was of prime importance.

The result of the project was clearly not a marketable product. The sensors were not reliable enough to be used by the patients, and the complete sensor suite and the ergometer in their current configuration would have been so expensive that a sustainable business model was out of reach at that point.

However, the results of the project were promising enough to exploit them in follow-up projects like OSAmI, which add additional use-cases for the setup and strive for a simplified configuration. Also the use of a service-oriented architecture together with broadly accepted, open standards helps to cope with the challenges that are described in this paper.

Acknowledgments The research leading to the results described in this paper has been funded in part by the European Community's Sixth Framework Programme under grant agreement IST 027074, SAPHIRE project, and in part by the German Federal Ministry of Education and Research (BMBF) under grant agreement 01 IS 08003, ITEA2 OSAmI project.

References

1. Dogac A, Laleci G, Kirbas S, Kabak Y, Sinir S, and Yildiz A. "Artemis: Deploying Semantically Enriched," in Web Services in the Healthcare Domain. Inf Syst J, special issue on Semantic Web and Web Services 2005.
2. Nee O, Gorath T, Hein A, Ludwig R, Willemsen D, Scheffold T, and Stahl K. "SAPHIRE: Ein System zur kardiologischen Tele-Rehabilitation," mdi—Forum der Medizin_Dokumentation und Medizin_Informatik, 2008;01:24–29.
3. Hein A, Nee O, Willemsen D, Scheffold T, Dogac A, and Laleci G. "SAPHIRE—Intelligent Healthcare Monitoring based on Semantic Interoperability Platform—The Homecare Scenario," in ECEH. 2006;191–202.
4. Dolin RH, Alschuler L, Boyer S, Beebe C, Behlen FM, Biron PV, and Shabo (Shvo) A, "HL7 Clinical Document Architecture, Release 2," J Am Med Inform Assoc. 2006;13(1):30–39. Available: http://www.jamia.org/cgi/content/abstract/13/1/30.
5. IHE, "Technical Framework Volume I Revision 5.0," Tech. Rep., August 2009, final Text. Available: http://www.ihe.net/Technical_Framework/upload/IHE_PCC_TF_5-0_Vol_1_2009-08-10.pdf.
6. Lohr KN, Field MJ, Committee On clinical practice guidelines, D. of health care services, and I. of medicine, guidelines for clinical practice : from development to use, Field MJ and Lohr KN, editors. National Academy Press, Washington, DC, 1992;1:45–54.
7. EU Directive 95/46/EC. Available: http://europa.eu.int/com-m/internal_market/privacy/law_en.htm.
8. Supplementary Directive 2002/58/EC. Available: http://europa.eu.int/information_society/topics/ecomm/useful_information/library/legislation/index_en. htm.
9. World Health Organization. Fact sheet N°317. Cardiovascular diseases (CVDs). 2009. Available: http://www.who.int/mediacentre/factsheets/fs317/en/print.html
10. Allender S, Scarborough P, Peto V, Rayner M, Leal J, Luengo-Fernandez R, and Gray A. "Heart network: European cardiovascular disease statistics", 2008. Available: http://swissheartgroups.ch/%5C/uploads/media/European_cardiovascular_disease_statistics_2008.pdf

11. Nobel JJ and Norman GK. "Emerging information management technologies and the future of disease management." Dis Manag. 2003;6(4):219–231. Available: 10.1089/109350703322682531.
12. Corrà U, Giannuzzi P, Adamopoulos S, Bjornstad H, Bjarnason-Weherns B, Cohen-Solal A, Dugmore D, Fioretti P, Gaita D, Hambrecht R, Hellermans I, McGee H, Mendes M, Perk J, Saner H, Vanhees L, Working Group On cardiac rehabilitation, and E. P. of the European society of cardiology, "Executive summary of the position paper of the Working Group on Cardiac Rehabilitation and Exercise Physiology of the European Society of Cardiology (ESC): core components of cardiac rehabilitation in chronic heart failure." Eur J Cardiovasc Prev Rehabil. 2005;12(4):321–325, Aug 2005.
13. Kotseva K, Wood D, Backer GD, Bacquer DD, Pyörälä K, Keil U, and E. U. R. O. A. S. P. I. R. E. S. Group, "EUROASPIRE III: a survey on the lifestyle, risk factors and use of cardioprotective drug therapies in coronary patients from 22 European countries." Eur J Cardiovasc Prev Rehabil. 2009;16(2):121–137, Apr 2009. Available: 10.1097/HJR.0b013e3283294b1d.
14. de Werf FV, Ardissino D, Betriu A, Cokkinos DV, Falk E, Fox KAA, Julian D, Lengyel M, Neumann F-J, Ruzyllo W, Thygesen C, Underwood SR, Vahanian A, Verheugt FWA, Wijns W, and Task Force On the management of acute myocardial infarction of the European Society of Cardiology, "Management of acute myocardial infarction in patients presenting with ST-segment elevation. The task force on the management of acute myocardial infarction of the European Society of Cardiology." Eur Heart J. 2003;24(1):28–66, Jan 2003.
15. Smith SC, Allen J, Blair SN, Bonow RO, Brass LM, Fonarow GC, Grundy SM, Hiratzka L, Jones D, Krumholz HM, Mosca L, Pasternak RC, Pearson T, Pfeffer MA, Taubert KA, A. H. A. C. C., L. National Heart, and B. Institute, "AHA/ACC guidelines for secondary prevention for patients with coronary and other atherosclerotic vascular disease: 2006 update: endorsed by the National Heart, Lung, and Blood Institute." Circulation. 2006;113(19):2363–2372, May 2006.
16. Völler H, Hahmann H, Gohlke H, Klein G, Rombeck B, Binting S, and Willich SN, "gerEffects of inpatient rehabilitation on cardiovascular risk factors in patients with coronary heart disease. PIN-Study Group," gerDtsch Med Wochenschr. 1999;124(27):817–823, Jul 1999. Available: 10.1055/s-2007-1024425.
17. Nee O and Hein A, "Clinical decision support with guidelines and bayesian networks," in decision support systems advances. In: Devlin G, Editor INTECH, 2010 pp. 117–136.
18. Busch C, Baumbach C, Willemsen D, Nee O, Gorath T, Hein A, and Scheffold T, "Supervised training with wireless monitoring of ECG, blood pressure and oxygen-saturation in cardiac patients." J Telemed Telecare. 2009. 15(3):112–114. Available: 10.1258/jtt.2009.003002.
19. Dissemination plans of the SAPHIRE project prepared by ALTEC, "http://www.srdc.metu.edu.tr/webpage/projects/saphire/index.php?option=com_content&view=article&id=57&Itemid=58," Tech. Rep.
20. Microsoft Corporation. Devices Profile for Web Services. 2006. Available: http://specs.xmlsoap.org/ws/2006/-02/devprof/devicesprofile.pdf.
21. Lipprandt M, Eichelberg M, Thronicke W, Kruger J, Druke I, Willemsen D, Busch C, Fiehe C, Zeeb E, and Hein A, "OSAMI-D: an open service platform for healthcare monitoring applications,"In: Proceedindgs 2nd Conference on Human System Interaction HSI '09. 2009;139–145.
22. Klompmaker F, Nebe K, Busch C, and Willemsen D, "Designing context aware user interfaces for online exercise training supervision," In: Proceedings of the 2nd Conference on Human System Interactions HSI'09. Piscataway, NJ, USA: IEEE Press, 2009;129–132.
23. Eichelberg M, Stewing F-J, Thronicke W, Hackbarth K, Seufert M, Busch C, Hein A, Krumm H, Ditze M, and Golatowski F. "OSAMI Commons: Eine Softwareplattform für flexible verteilte Dienstesysteme über Geräten und eingebetteten Systemen," in 2. Deutscher AAL-Kongress. 2009 vol. 2. Berlin: VDE, January pp. 269–272.
24. Jovanov E, Milenkovic A, Otto C, Groen PD, Johnson B, Warren S, and Taibi G, "A WBAN system for ambulatory monitoring of physical activity and health status: applications and challenges." Conference Proceedings IEEE Eng Med Biol Soc. 2005;4:3810–3813. Available: 10.1109/IEMBS.2005.1615290.

An Intelligent Multi-Agent Memory Assistant

Ângelo Costa and Paulo Novais

Abstract World population is ageing and increasingly scarce resources are required to cover the needs of everyone adequately. Medical conditions, especially memory problems, restrict the daily life of a broad slice of the elderly population, affect their independence. To prevent this, providing the right care and assistance while having in mind the costs implicated is essential. One possible path is to work with resources that we already have today and create innovative solutions to achieve the required level of support. There are not many solutions either technological or not to prevent memory loss. In this work we present a possible solution aimed at restoring or maintaining the independence of elderly people, through the use of so-called Memory Assistants. We thus present an Intelligent Multi-Agent Memory Assistant designed to help people with memory problems remember their events and activities. The implementation of an event manager, free time manger, medication remainder and a sensory system, to manage and monitor the user, we aim to improve their quality of life and increase their independence.

Keywords Ambient assisted living · Memory assistants · Monitoring · Multi-agent system · Scheduling · Sensors

Â. Costa (✉) · P. Novais
Departamento de Informática, Universidade do Minho, Braga, Portugal
e-mail: acosta@di.uminho.pt

P. Novais
e-mail: pjon@di.uminho.pt

Commun Med Care Compunetics (2011) 3: 197–221
DOI: 10.1007/8754_2011_18
© Springer-Verlag Berlin Heidelberg 2011
Published Online: 28 April 2011

1 Introduction

How will our life be when we get old?

We pose this question in our daily life almost every day. The answer is: there is no answer. In fact, each technological evolution adds another variable to our possible future. At most we, as Humans, envision a future that is not too broad or too restricted. The technology that surrounds us changes our life for better or for worse. In fact, if we look back 20 years, the computer field was complex and restricted to trained engineers and technicians. Nowadays, even a child can efficiently operate a computer. Thus, it is not wrong to say that our life is shaped by technological evolution. Going along this flow, the elderly community is now prone to accept new technologies and is in fact prepared to work with new devices.

1.1 Motivation

The last census made by the United Nations revealed that most of the European developed countries show a decreasing rate of new-borns and, at the same time, are the ones with a greater percentage of elderly persons, as can be seen in Fig. 1. This phenomenon is also seen in several other developed countries around the globe. The main causes that can be pointed out are the quality of current health-care services and better and healthier life styles. At the same time, these countries also having now a culture oriented to have fewer children, with these children having a better quality of life [1].

The provision of social services, especially health care, to a growing percentage of elderly is not attainable in the future with the structure of current society. It is our main objective to provide an answer to typical problems that arise in people when they are in an elderly stage. The social implications imply a response to the problem.

In our perspective, the answer must be a sustainable solution, economic and socially, supported by technology—electronic devices and computer applications. We propose a solution based on devices fairly cheap that can provide several features in a small and discrete manner. The adoption of a technological solution means that the persons that will benefit from it, the elderly ones, can have access to it with small costs involved, and because it is a combination of software and hardware, upgrades and new features are easier to implement.

1.2 Aging Factors

With age, memory problems tend to arise. Recent studies show that we tend to start having memory losses at around 50 years of age [2, 3], with a trend to worsen

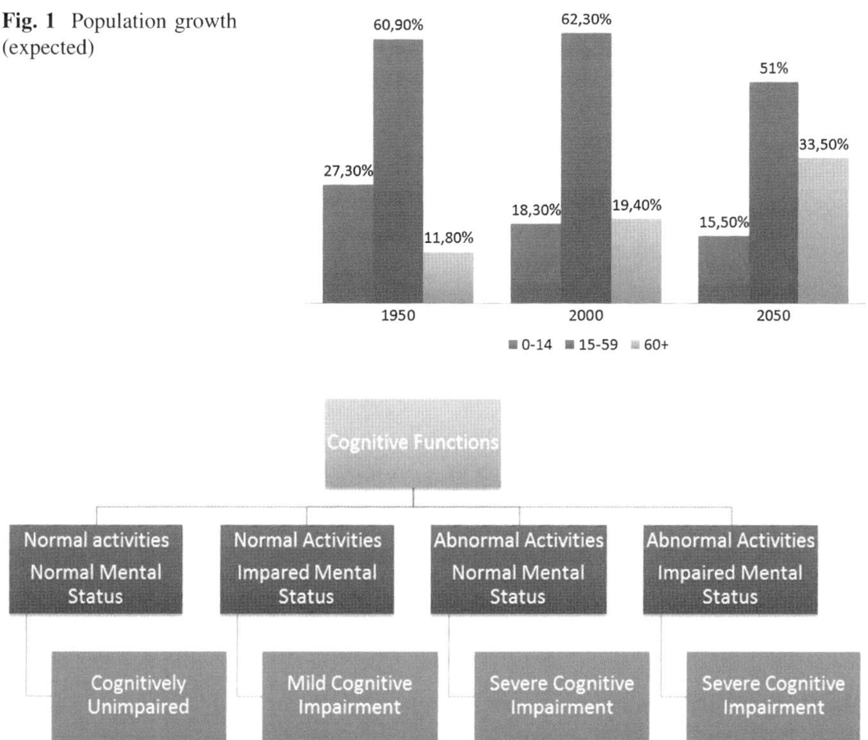

Fig. 2 Memory degeneration steps [4]

as age increases. In the path to total memory loss, several stages can be identified. The stages are well known in the psychology and medical areas and are depicted in Fig. 2 [4]. To determine the current stage of a particular patient, practitioners generally rely on tests performed to that patient. The results of the tests are then compared to the ones of a regular person, and a diagnosis is achieved. These tests consist in routines, questions and activities related to the user, organized in two common groups: comprehensive tests and brainwave analysis. There are three possible outcomes: cognitively impaired (normal daily experiences), mild cognitive impairment (daily life experiences mildly affected) and severe cognitive impairment (needs constant supervision).

MCI, or Memory Cognitive Impairment, is the measure of the memory loss steps. The bigger the index, the worse the condition of the patient. Figure 3 depicts the evolution of the disease in the United States [5]. In this figure, it can be seen that there is an increase of 200% in 10 years only.

Currently, modern societies are not prepared to give support to the increased elderly population, although some have cultural behaviours that advocate the care of the elderly. Nevertheless, at this moment, virtually every country urgently needs innovative solutions and approaches to accommodate and take care of the elderly.

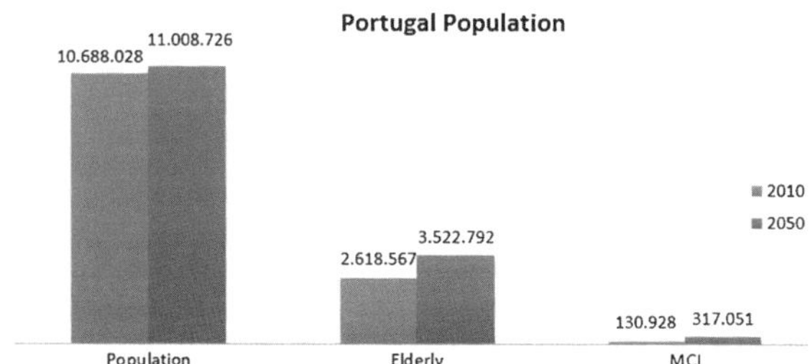

Fig. 3 Graph of the expected evolution of MCI in the Portuguese population

1.3 Possible Paths

Given the urgency of the problem, there is a need for approaches that can be tested and implemented presently and available to full use in a near future. The services available nowadays to help elderly in their daily tasks are very scarce and are not nearly as focused on the actual problems as they should.

The development of technological solutions that make an integrated use of these already existing services is the best approach. In fact, software and hardware solutions are the best way to easily improve and implement tools to assist the users essentially because they are relatively cheap, easy to upgrade, fully configurable and adaptable, and allow the implementation of new functionalities.

In terms of already developed solutions to the memory problems, the medical community essentially suggests [6] the use of games and tests to enhance the patient's brain activity and the implementation of activities that break everyday routines. As an example, tests and playful activities are now used as part of the treatment to Alzheimer's disease. This disease still has no known cure and the best that can be done is to prevent or slow down the loss of the remaining mental abilities [7].

Another important fact, revealed by a study carried on the University of Harvard [6] is that the part of the brain that we use to store the long term memories is also responsible for the creation of new thoughts and ideas, an ability commonly known as *envisioning*. Consequently, the loss of saved memories has as one of its consequences a decrease in the ability to project new activities. Another problem is the loss of a simple and very common skill: *the cause and consequence*. This ability is what tells us that doing a given task will probably have a given outcome, by having done a similar task in the past or by simple logic. An example can be: when opening a faucet, water will pour through that faucet. This is a simple example but it causes impact in our everyday life. Without this skill, whenever a new complex task is learned, for example by viewing another person executing it, in the next day the patient will not be able to infer the consequences of its execution, if requested to.

1.4 VirtualECare Project

1.4.1 Ambient Assisted Living

Ambient Assisted Living (AAL) is a relatively new paradigm that emerged in the 1980s. It is a junction of domotics with intelligent and proactive software applications, aimed at implementing intelligent systems inside common domestic environments, in order to assist the patient and control the environment and the devices around him [7].

AAL is currently an active topic of research, with new projects arising to complete previous ones or to present new functionalities that were not developed before. Actually, the AAL paradigm can take several forms, shaping itself according to the devices at the user's home or even attached to/in the user's body, to fully fledge top-level projects [23].

1.4.2 VirtualECare Objectives

The VirtualECare project (VEC) focuses on a high-level view of the Ambient Assisted Living field. It assures the complete panoply of services to aid and assist elderly persons or people in need. It spans all the layers ranging from the user and the sensors in his home environment, to high level Group Decision Support Systems. It aims at a complete solution to a fairly recent and under-explored problem: the provision of health-care services directly at the home of the elderly [8].

VEC is also acting as an enabler for complementary smaller-level projects, being developed on the basis of service-sharing and functionality complementarity. One of them deals with the implementation of sensors in an environment, aimed at monitoring its users and acquiring important information, in order to create and refine an individual profile for each one of the known users. The project started with an initial implementation of a simulation platform that could either realistically simulates sensors or actually be connected to real ones. Having received a positive feedback from the scientific community, the project is under on-going development to implement several other interesting features. Specifically, researchers are now dealing with the determination of the user's mood and with the challenge of connecting this platform with other higher level projects, such as the VEC (Fig. 4).

In terms of core functionalities, the data collected is used to adjust the actions and decisions implemented in the user typical profile in order to comply more accurately with the user needs. The profiles are very important as they are useful to create an initial picture of the user's typical preferences. In fact, personalization is an important feature for two main reasons: it allows achieving better resources assignment and higher levels of user comfort.

In terms of resources assignment, the system should be able to, through the use of a personalization map, infer what feature is most important and what actions are best to execute, in order to respond to specific problems. If the user likes a room colder than the usually programmed, the system should take into account that

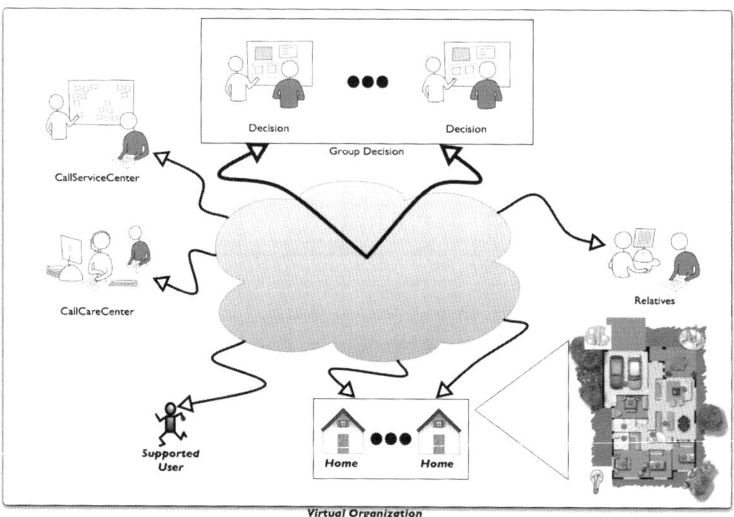

Fig. 4 VirtualECare areas of interest

information since the first day of implementation. This is also useful in scenarios in which there is a conflict of user's definitions, which happens when two or more users are in the same room and have different needs or preferences, with the system having to reach a compromise between both of the user definitions.

In terms of user's comfort, the system should be able to take decisions not in a generic way but in a rather focused one. The ability of taking actions that were carefully adjusted to the user is important so that the user does not have to correct the system periodically. In this sense, it is also important that the system has the mechanisms to determine if the user has special conditions (e.g. physical impairments) and adjust its actions accordingly.

The memory assistant area is very recent and some projects arise with the objective to solve inherent social problems that are clearly identified [7]. In fact most of the current developments have many flaws. Whilst the social problems are clearly identified, the solutions aren't, and this means that the solutions that are available, although in the core functions giving an answer to the detected problems, are not well accepted by the community that will be using them. The *form following function* of the projects available nowadays have to be heavily reconsidered. For instance, most of the projects available to an elderly community do not have visual interfaces that cope with usual imparities that are common at an older age. Other common situation is that applications and projects are made by younger people, and it is our opinion that they do not have the real perception of how the world is viewed and operated by an elderly person. In the memory assistants' area these problems are heavily amplified, and being such a broad area, the projects are scarce and spread apart. As being a part of the AAL, the memory assistants have a large area of operation, this means that there are benefits as well problems, such as providing different solutions to different questions, but not having a streamlined solution and interpretation of each question means that every project can provide a solution unique from each other, and any of them cannot respond correctly to the user demands.

This document is organized as follows: Sect. 2 describes the Memory assistants' area and other related projects. Section 3 the technical overview. Section 4 presents the architecture and the several modules of this project. In Sect. 5 the application scenarios and results of the tests, and finally, Sect. 6 shows the conclusions and future work.

2 Memory Assistants

The memory assistants' area is a fairly new one, thus having innovative solutions to new problems. This also means that the projects available are very recent and have very different focus on the direction the solutions should be really heading. A presentation of different projects that are populating the memory assistants' area follows, exposing their features and flaws.

2.1 *HERMES*

HERMES [9] is a project developed together by CURE-Center for Usability Research and Engineering, INGEMA Foundation, IBM Haifa Research Lab, University of Bradford, Athens Information Technology and TXT e-Solutions. It is supported by the EU under the Framework Programme 7 and aims at providing an independent living and social participation to elderly persons, by improving the quality of life. The main objective is to develop software and hardware tools that will reduce the negative impact of declining cognitive capabilities, particularly the memory-related ones. An important feature of this project is the implementation of a monitoring system which should be able to record every action and associated choices of one user. This will later be used to build a map of associations of the different events and, based on that map, create a pattern that emulates the human memory mechanisms.

Despite its ambitious goals, HERMES is still in a very early stage of development. Thus, the developed tools are still very simple, with low effectiveness and an amount of problems that have no known time of resolution. For instance, the speech recording tool must be executed in certain limited parameters in order for the speech to be converted to text and the system still needs to be manually trained for each user.

2.2 *SenseCam*

SenseCam [10] is basically a wearable camera that passively records photos, without the user's intervention. The objective is to report, through images, the user's daily activities and the places he has been to. The hardware contains even some degree of automation, e.g. light-intensity and light colour sensors, body heat detector and motion sensors. It was designed to be used as a pendant on a necklace but it may also be clipped in pockets or belts, or attached in clothing. The key idea is that the user, at the end of the day or on a posterior day can remember his past activities by watching the pictures taken while doing them.

Although the Microsoft Research Center claims it is a memory assistant for elderly, it has in fact no significant on-the-fly abilities for reminding its users of events and/or tasks. It is merely a so-called time machine, like a video camera used to record what the user has done. However, it serves the purpose of remembering what the user he/she has done, in a specific time or day. It has not any kind of associated intelligence and it is merely useful for users with total memory loss, like Alzheimer's.

2.3 M4L: Memories for Life

Developed by the Engineering and Physical Sciences Research Council (EPSRC), United Kingdom, M4L has as objective to use technological solutions to assist the user's memory [11]. This project focuses on five different fields: health, private life, education, entertainment and science.

Currently it is proposed as a raw data archive centre with a significant capacity. This way, it can store a wide range of information about every user. The access to the data can be performed by handheld devices or computers that have a constant connection to the server. The healthcare field is currently designed to store all clinical information about the user. The private life field consists in saving all the items that are dear to the user, like his photos or financial data for example. The education, entertainment and science fields have as aim to save all the data available so that it can later be processed and selected by the user. The end result is an attempt to eliminate all the paper used nowadays and, at the same time, interconnect all the people involved in a seamless way. As it is currently used as an undifferentiated memory bank, the objective is to make a collection of well selected memories of the user.

As the project is still in a research and implementation phase, the current results are somewhat disappointing. Basically, what is holding this project back is the large amount of storage space needed for maintaining all this information. Thus, significant and practical breakthroughs are only expected in the long term, as the price of storage decreases.

The projects presented are valid in essence but miss some points. From a high level point of view, it may be said that the main problems are these: in the case of the SenseCam the problem is interactivity; in the case of Hermes is the ability to map all the necessary connections and the resources available; and in the case of M4L is the storage and retrieval of major information.

With very different scopes the presented projects stand apart from each other, namely the HERMES project from the other ones. The HERMES project was a solid and futuristic point of view of the possible conceptions that should be available to the user. Also the complexity is at a completely different level, involving computer science and medical science, namely the neuroscience. The same cannot be applied to the other presented projects that are more simplistic but their goals are easily achievable.

3 Technology Overview

This section presents an overview of the technologies used in this project. The following descriptions underline their use, how they shape the way the project is constructed and its behaviour, and the benefits from its usage.

3.1 Multi-Agent Systems

From our point of view, the best paradigm that can fulfil the development requisites of Memory Assistants is the Multi-Agent System one [12]. The use of MAS in the development of an application platform enables modularity, expansibility, standardization, platform independence and the implementation of intelligent behaviours (e.g. negotiation, argumentation). Generally, agent platforms support the interaction between the agents by means of communication protocols and standards, facilitating the development process and laying the path for cross-platform compatibility. Intelligent agents can work in collaboration or individually, depending on their goals.

Agents can also be completely decentralized and are typically independent from each other. Given their flexibility, agents are easy to restructure and modify without having to change the entire platform or even having to change the communication methods. Well-developed communication ontology at the beginning of the project allows the system to use it for several functions, even if the agents are changed along the way. The implementation will follow the Wooldridge and Jennings definition of strong agent [13], an agent that is generally referred to as a computer system that is either conceptualized or implemented using concepts that are more usually applied to humans.

The fault-tolerance provided by the MAS is also crucial. If an agent has problems, the platform can continue to operate, even if at that time the services provided by that agent are not available. This can be solved by launching a new agent to take over the operations of the one that failed, given that the state of the agents is maintained outside the scope of the agents.

Another important characteristic for the development of a software platform is the possibility to develop the agents in offline mode, i.e., agents can be constructed in a replicated platform that operates in an offline mode. If they pass the stability tests, they can be launched without any loss in the main platform. The use of a MAS is one of the main characteristics of this project as it shapes its architecture. All the functionalities are provided by agents, thus the system inherits all the characteristics mentioned above.

3.2 JADE

The JADE Framework is an elegant and simple way to develop a MAS. Working over the JAVA platform means that it benefits from the use of object-oriented programming, has a large developing community and can be ported to virtually any hardware. The JADE Framework is already well-known to the Intelligent Systems and Artificial Intelligence fields, with significant projects relying on its use [14].

3.3 Communications

The communication layer is also supported by the JADE Framework. It follows a strict ontology, with the content expressed in XML language. The use of XML guarantees both human and machine readability and the correct tagging and field processing. The content is encrypted and is transferred in messages that rely on the HTTP protocol.

The proposed platform is a distributed one, so it is essential to provide the necessary mechanisms for cooperation and coordination in order to allow the agents to proceed correctly with their tasks. In that sense, the communication between the several existing agents can be established over several protocols, namely Ethernet, WIFI, GSM and UMTS. Moreover, the communication protocol complies with FIPA's (Foundation for Intelligent Physical Agents) Agent Communication Language (ACL).

3.4 Prolog

The Prolog computing language is a logic inferential one. This type of programming guarantees the mathematical treatment needed in the decision processes implemented. With the use of Prolog, which is a mathematical logical language, there is the absolute certainty of the outcome of the functions. As it is rooted in formal language it takes advantage in being correct, fast and easy to implement, thus making the decision easier to implement and fault proof.

3.5 Android

With the adoption of JAVA/JADE, the development and implementation of the tools and interfaces in mobile devices, namely the Android-based ones, is easy and seamless. The implementation of distributed memory assistants in mobile devices is an advantage as users gain mobility and can make use of the functionalities provided independently of the location. An advantage of the Android platform over the others available mobile platforms (iOS, Windows Mobile, Blackberry OS, etc.) is that is open-source and it is free and easy to develop new applications.

4 iGenda: A Multi-Agent Memory Assistant

The depicted social problems, the fact that there are unfocused resources and the assumption that current projects are not providing quite the expected solution or having no actual implementation, constituted the motivation for the start of the iGenda project. This was one of the projects that emerged out of the VEC, and that was interesting enough to be decoupled and developed stand-alone, although in cooperation.

This project intends to be a response to a gap in the still undeveloped memory assistant field. This being a relatively new field, several application scenarios can be envisioned. One of them is its use in a hospital environment to improve the physician routines and clinical duties, also connecting the patients, whether they are in the hospital or in their homes [15]. Another possible scenario is its use of active body sensors to register the vital signs in order to monitor the user's health condition and schedule, in both user's and physician's agendas, an appointment and an event. Ultimately, the system should be sufficiently autonomous to request an urgent medical response. In fact, the modular nature of the iGenda architecture allows using the same base architecture and extending it to such application scenarios, through service and functionalities reuse [16]. And, an important point is that this can be done without interfering with the functionalities that are already implemented.

As the projects presented in this field are scarce, this is our effort to accomplish the objectives proposed and fill this gap. Our objective is to apply the above presented memory assistant under a new vision, the intelligent agendas [17].

Moreover, we are also concerned with the patients and their relatives as the social support is of utter importance, mainly in the cases of elderly living alone. Therefore, the iGenda allows patient's relatives or friends to register as users of the system, to be able to access information about the patient. For example, a relative of the user can login to see when the next appointment is scheduled. The sharing of events is also supported among the group of users of a patient. In that sense, it is possible to create shared calendars and activities that are public to users of the group, incorporating this information into the agendas already being used by the users seamlessly.

In this section we highlight its architecture and main modules.

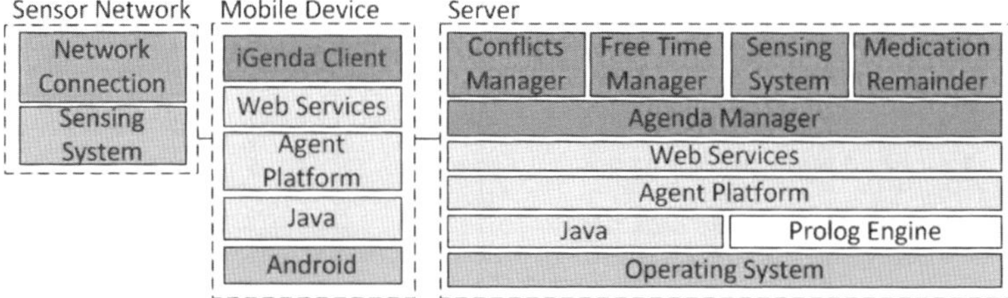

Fig. 5 The iGenda architecture

4.1 Architecture

The architecture of iGenda is based on the agent paradigm [18]. Every core action has an individual agent to support the activity and the decision, as it can be seen in Fig. 5. This way, it is safer and more immune to possible flaws. And, should they appear, it is easier to track them down and correct the problem.

The architecture presented in Fig. 5 represents a multi-platform project. The server will create most of the decisions, the system being used to provide a mobile interface to the user and serve for the connection to the sensor system. In the figure are depicted the different operating systems, interpreters and agents. The agents assure the decision and establish the communications between the remaining agents and platforms.

All the decisions are independent logic implementations. These logic implementations are done in Constraint Logic Programming, which means that there is a close proximity with the logic rules. This approach translates in the types of predicates being taken into account as affirmations of truth. The affirmations are then tested accordingly to the algorithms implemented: if they fit, the test is successful; otherwise, the predicates are negated. This approach translates into a broad acceptance of predicates and variables, not being restricted to one input only. In lay terms, the algorithms are not a cadence of "ifs", but are "if-not", the inversion means that more tests can be made, not stressing the system by using a large amount of tests.

At the beginning of the project this approach was not implemented and, very often, tests failed because if the result was not as expected, the logic engines could not process them, thus narrowing the spectrum of cases that could be processed.

The agents may communicate over different protocols (e.g. Ethernet, WIFI, GSM, and UMTS, among others). The communication protocol complies with the FIPA-ACL standard, using JADE as the agent platform and the protocol XMLCodec for coding the content (Fig. 6). All the agents are compliant with the ACL standard. Moreover, agents were also developed in JADE-Leap so that they can be implemented on mobile devices with limited resources. The support of the Health Level Seven International standard (HL7) is also a feature to be implemented, as the direct connection to hospitals is in study. This well established language will provide bidirectional communications between the institutions and the iGenda.

Fig. 6 Communication
workflow

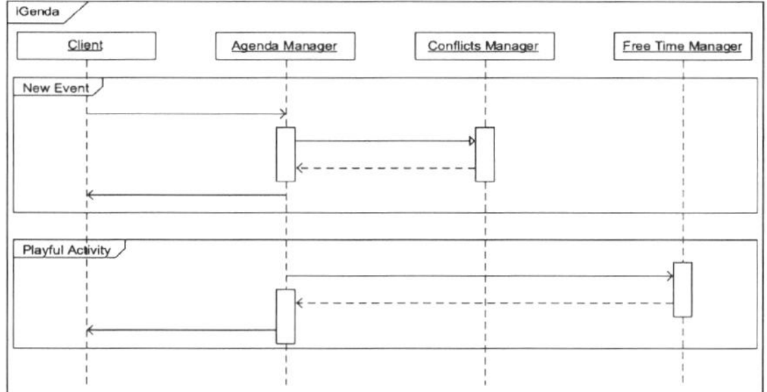

Initially, the project had only a little part dedicated to mobile devices. The approach was to have a mobile terminal that communicated with the user to notify him of the most important tasks. Now, as the project evolves, it is clear that a great deal of the functionalities must somehow be supported by mobile devices. This is enabled by seamless and location-independent connectivity to networks and enhanced computational features, such as GPS and sensors availability. Moreover, as it can be seen in the description of the remaining modules (Fig. 7), the mobile device is currently the best alternative to make the bridge between the users and the actual application: it is always present, it is lightweight, and it is always connected. This also represents a shift from a centric architecture to a distributed one, in which the emphasis is placed on the user nodes, making the application closer to the personal context of its users.

4.1.1 Core Modules

The iGenda is not a static system common to every user as each user has its own personalized iGenda instance, as seen in Fig. 8. In the development of this project, a centralized management encompassing all users was not considered as it brings problems concerning scaling, performance and stability. The independent processing of each user is more reliable and, if an instance of iGenda crashes, it only crashes one user platform while the remaining keeps running. This approach also makes it easier to process the incoming connections and to manage the authorized users that can access the main user calendar. Let us now depict the core modules that make up the iGenda architecture.

Agenda Manager

The Agenda Manager (AM) connects and controls the conflicts manager system and the scheduling system, using the communication infrastructure available to receive and send requests. As a result, the AM is responsible for the communication and security of the whole platform.

In that sense, the AM is the communication gateway. It can assume either a passive execution mode or a dominant one, depending on its configuration or demands.

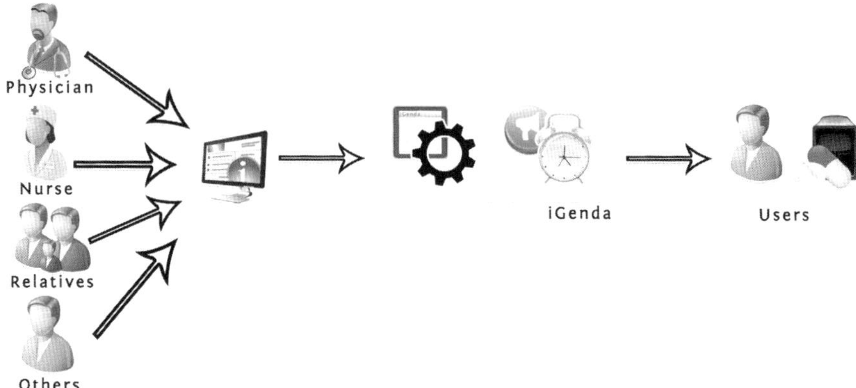

Fig. 7 A high level view of iGenda

Fig. 8 One iGenda for each
user

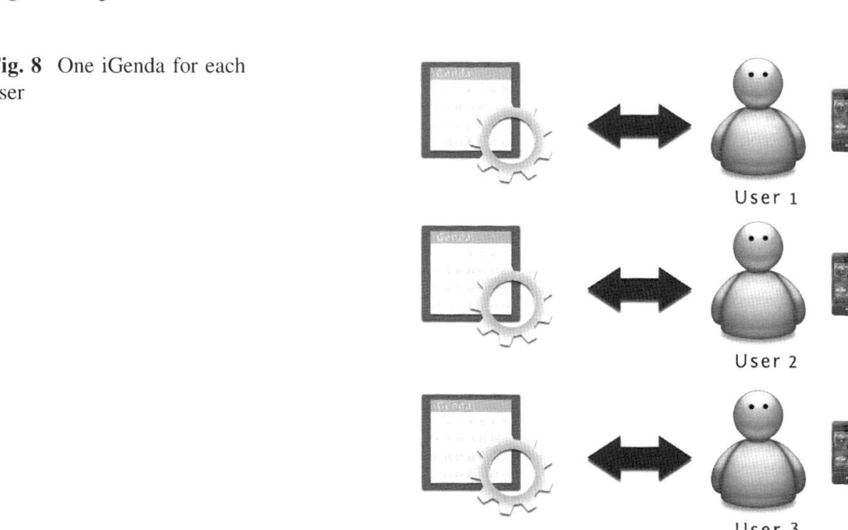

The passive mode constitutes the standard execution mode. In this mode, messages can be received and processed, and respond properly to the involving agents. In the dominant mode, the AM controls the other user's iGenda sub-platforms. This agent is configured directly on the agenda and sends demanding messages to the iGenda's users (Fig. 8). The AM also ensures that the user's friends and relatives are in touch and know what activities he is or will be doing in the near future.

Conflicts Manager

The Conflicts Manager (CM) agent has as main objective to ensure that there is no overlap of activities and events. This module schedules or reorganizes each event ensuring that it is in accordance with the remaining ones. The CM is essentially a sleeping agent that only activates when the AM sends him a message. His task is to receive the incoming messages and process them.

The agent is divided into two main parts: the JAVA component receives the messages containing a potential new appointment and respective content to process while the logic engine decides how that appointment should be scheduled, taking into consideration factors like other appointments and respective priorities. When a new appointment arrives, several tests are done by the logic engine in order to determine the position in the agenda in which it should be placed. At this moment, 16 different tests are performed to see if the events fit. For instance the simplest test available is the one that verifies if an event fits in an empty space, or if it collides with existing events.

Each event received comes with an associated priority value. This value is attributed either by the user that is scheduling it or by the system. In the cases in which it is the user setting up a new high priority event, his role is verified to determine if he has the privileges to schedule that type of events. The priority values are numbered from 1 to 50, although it is not expected to the values to pass from 10. In this scale, a value of 1 denotes health-related events and is reserved to be used by physicians and medical staff only.

Given the complexity of dealing with temporal values, mainly due to the different units that compose a date value, the system uses a value in milliseconds instead of a traditional representation of a date. This makes time-related calculations much easier and gives a precision of milliseconds, rather than the precision of seconds of traditional date representation.

This process can be organized into three major steps: the initialization, the testing and the conclusion.

- Initialization: the CM JAVA component sends the calendar and the new event to the Prolog engine. This information contains all the activities to be executed in a period of time and additional information such as the priority of each activity or the persons involved.
- Testing: the Logic engine builds an internal interpretation of the calendar and tests the new event against the already scheduled ones. In the end, the outcome can be a new calendar if the process ends successfully or an error message otherwise.
- Conclusion: the Logic engine builds a new calendar and sends it back to the JAVA component, flagging it as complete, if the calendar was built successfully. Otherwise, it sends an error message that the JAVA component can interpret and notify the involved persons.

Free Time Manager

The main functionality of the Free Time Manager (FTM) is to schedule playful activities in the free time of the user. In fact, these activities are paramount for a healthy active aging as they promote culture, education and conviviality, based on an individualized plan.

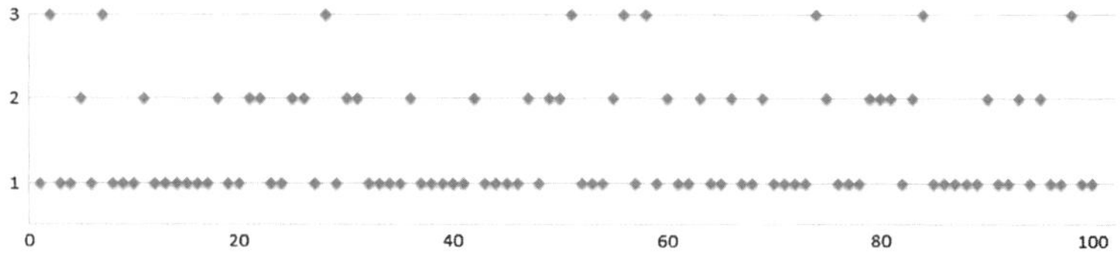

Fig. 9 Results of 100 tests and the chosen event

This agent can be fully configured to work in a way that maximizes each user's satisfaction. The FTM is activated by a trigger sent by the AM; this trigger is activated when its configured time is achieved. The process is relatively simple: the logic engine selects a possible action from a database using an algorithm that normalizes the choices and introduces a level of randomness to ensure that it does not always do the same choice.

Free Time Manager choosing function:

$$prio = \left\{ m_{prio} \ldots n_{prio} \right\}$$

$$a = \sum_{i=m_{prio}}^{n_{prio}} i$$

$$b = \sum_{i=1}^{m_{prio}} i$$

$$f(prio) = -1 * Rand(a) * b$$

$$(1)$$

In Fig. 9, the dots represent the activity selected, out of a group of 3 possibilities, as it can be seen, the activity 1 has the most hits, but the other activities are also selected along the way.

As mentioned before, each event has a priority value, which is also considered by the algorithm, represented in Eq. 1. The events selected are the ones that can fit the free space in the calendar. The *prio* series contain the events and the correspondent priority values; a is the sum of the priority all the possible events; b is the sum of all the possible events; and *Rand* is the function that results a random number in the a range.

Additional characteristics like overhead time (e.g. time to travel from current location of appointment location) are also described in the new activity so that the logic agent can accurately determine the time it takes to prepare an activity. The Logic module handles a large database of available activities and it does a selection of available events that can fit the available space. The selection algorithm picks one activity, and that event is saved in the calendar. This task is done for each free space, so multiple iterations are done in each execution.

4.1.2 Interface

In terms of the user interface, a basic one has been initially developed, merely to test the functionalities and the agent's interactions. This first interface is now going

Fig. 10 Snapshot from the
deprecated user interface

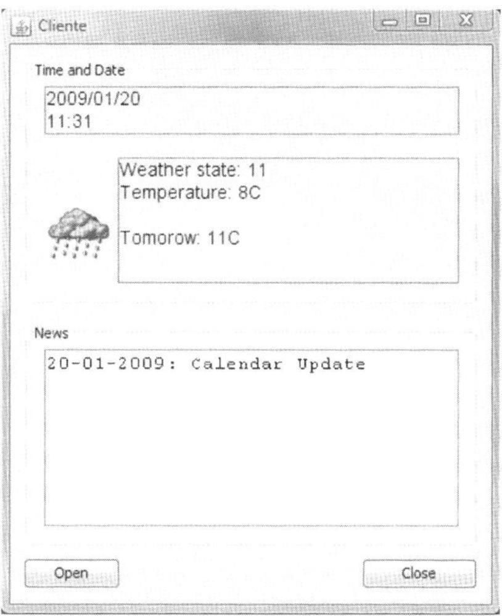

under major restructuring and was enriched with new visual and new functionalities, encompassing SMS and Voice Mail services. These two new functionalities
were developed mainly thinking of the elderly people who are not comfortable
with the use of more recent technological developments, so that technology does
not become a barrier. The deprecated user interface is shown in Fig. 10.

The new interface was developed according to a new paradigm: the use of
portable devices. The use of PDAs is the best way to grant portability and mobility
to the application, allowing the user to move freely and, nonetheless, continue
monitored and connected to the system. The new mobile interface can be seen in
Fig. 11.

The interface was developed to be similar to standard Android interfaces so that
users can quickly familiarize with it. In that sense, the learning curve of iGenda is
reduced. The main objective was to have an intuitive interface that flows under the
fingers of the user and that requires little or no training to use.

It is important to refer that the typical users should be used to operate devices
such as PDA's, or require a minimal amount of training and adaptation. The
Adaptive User Interface (AUI) is also an interesting feature to be added in a short
term period. It consists on creating interfaces that can be adjusted to the user needs
and preferences in terms of visualization and context. Given the target population
of this project, the solutions given by the AUI are fairly interesting to serve
correctly the results of the user, the way they were meant to be interpreted. Being
an engineer, the developer sometimes forgets that the user can only work with the
interface provided and this is a core factor, and at the same level as all the modules
and logical engines. But, as referred before, the target population being an elderly
one, we must not forget that there are also various problems that affect commonly
the elderly population. Problems like loss of vision and hearing are also very common at an older age, and interfaces provided by the operating system of the mobile
devices are not ready for those problems. Studies being done [19] in the visual and

Fig. 11 New android
interface

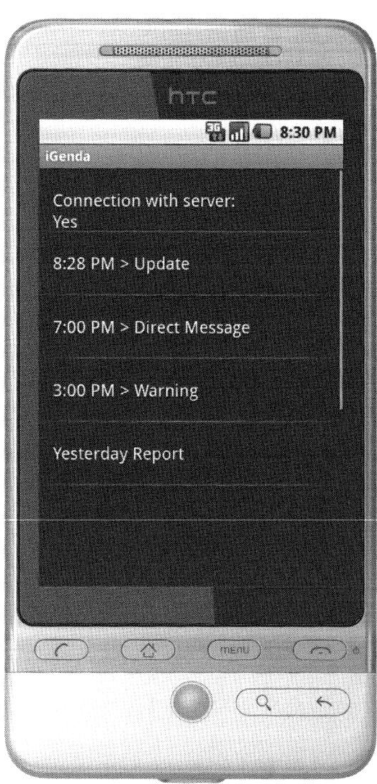

hearing problems suggest interfaces that provide, among other solutions, a high font
resolution and audio/voice commands.

The tests made by projects that solve problems in the referred areas, using
computer applications, report bad results when used by persons that are less
computer literate and substantial improvements when the users are used to operate
computers, even if they have vision and/or hearing impairments. The roadmap of
our project includes modular interfaces and pre-recorded commands, such as
voicemails, to notify the users of the activities to perform. It is not our main
objective to provide more advanced interfaces, such as active voice commands, as
the main focus of the project is a technical solution, the interfaces being provided
as clear and simple as possible. We recognise the fact that the acceptance by the
users can rely solely on the interface presented, but in an initial phase computer
literate users will be our main users. This is done so they can surpass the possible
interface problems and test the remaining modules of the iGenda system.

4.2 Medication Reminder

One of the worst consequences of memory impairments is a patient not remembering to take his drugs at the right time, or not remembering it at all. In that sense,
a Medication Reminder module was developed. It consists of three agents that

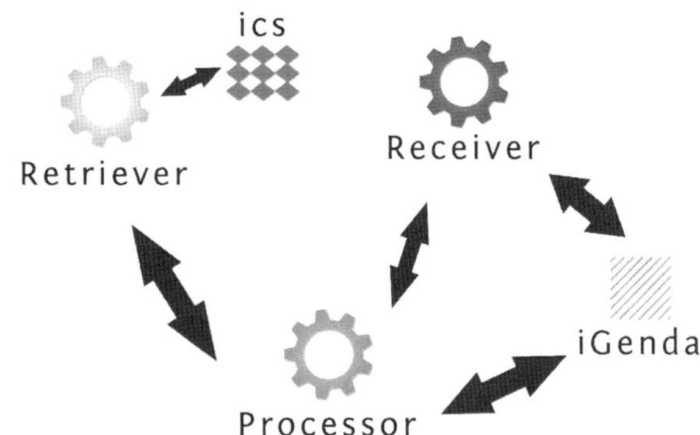

Fig. 12 Medication reminder platform

remind the user of the drugs he has to take, at the right time. Although this is apparently a simple problem, it is not so trivial to implement. Specifically, the agents consider the time to take the medication and the possible event of the user leaving the home, in which case an early notification must be issued in order for the patient to take the drugs with him. This module was developed independently rather than being integrated into the main iGenda application for two main reasons. The first is that the action of taking drugs is usually very brief and, thus, there is no need to schedule an event. The second reason is that the notifications should be different than the normal ones, with a higher degree of importance or urgency.

This module relies on 3 agents (Fig. 12): the Receiver, the Processor and the Retriever, with its functionalities as follows. The Receiver receives new schedules of drugs that must be taken by the user. This is done directly by the healthcare provider. The Retriever fetches the upcoming drug-related events and puts them in memory so that the Processor can perform correctly: it is the bridge between the database and the Processor. Finally, the Processor receives the information delivered by the Retriever and warns the user when the right time comes, prepares the next warning.

4.3 Sensing System

The Sensing System is a module that interfaces with sensors used directly on the user, acquiring information from his vital signs and health status [20]. This module can detect and prevent any issues that may threaten the health of the user, as it can detect problems that are occurring in real time. In fact, acquiring information about the patient's vital signs is the fastest and more reliable way to assess his health status. Therefore, it allows the system to know if the patient is under stress or in danger and also if he is able to perform the events scheduled. It also opens the door to intelligent and proactive scheduling. This means that, in a scenario in which the patient's health status is deteriorating over time, the Sensing System can connect to the iGenda and ask for an automatic scheduling of a potentially urgent medical

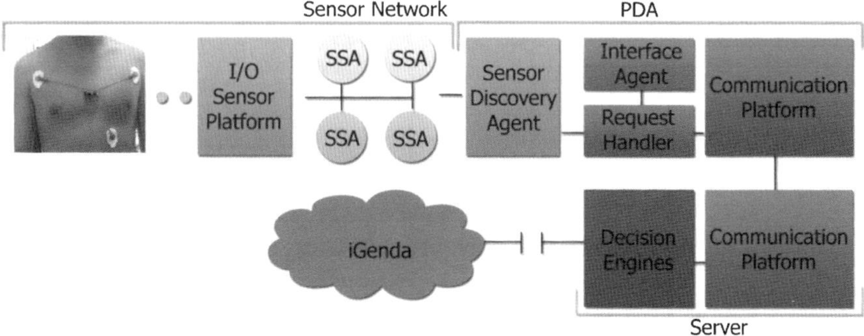

Fig. 13 The current architecture of the sensing system

appointment. The iGenda schedules the request in both the patient's and physician's agendas.

Moreover, this sensing system also makes use of GPS sensors, possibly available in the mobile device. The key idea is to have access to the current location of the user for two main purposes: determine travel overheads for efficient response in case of emergency.

This module is constituted by several sensors that capture the patient's vital signs, electrocardiogram, blood pressure, oximetry and temperature, processes them in order to be readable for Humans. From this point on, the data is interpreted and the system configured to read the data and, by means of well-defined clinical guidelines, trigger appropriate actions if necessary.

Currently, the sensing system in an advanced stage of development (Fig. 13), having already a beta version constituted by both software and hardware modules. It thus collects data for processing and interpreting the health status in order to create rules that can be used by the iGenda Core to better implement, schedule and manage the user's daily life and respective activities.

4.4 Centralized Management System

The main objective of the Centralized Management System (CMS) is to create a super iGenda system that supports multi-person scheduling and multi-layer calendars [21, 22]. It is being developed to work in medical environments such as hospitals and should not be seen as a sub-module of iGenda but rather as a fork.

The main objective is to control the routines of physicians and nurses and device functionalities to achieve:

- Better health provision;
- Higher control of time spent in each task;
- Improved routing through tasks;
- Improved selection of patient's priority according to health status.

This module is currently under development. Therefore, we are currently studying different algorithms that can deal with several users and their respective roles and tasks, keeping in mind the above proposed objectives. In face of the problems of NP-Complete complexity we are currently facing, the solution will most likely consist of genetic algorithms. The complexity of the problems arises mostly because a single routine route usually requires more than one person. Given that Human resources tend to be limited and that each one has his own tasks, a significant work of optimization and coordination must be performed.

5 Application Scenarios

In this project there are two type scenarios: *single user* and *institution.*

The *single user* scenario is one in which the user has an iGenda platform and has the possibility to be connected either to a healthcare institution or directly to a physician. In this scenario, the platform is optimized to adjust to each user, to respond to the user's necessities.

The *institution* scenario corresponds to the description of the CMS module. The institution will have a set of objectives and practitioners, like physicians and nurses, will comply with the instructions given by the CMS platform. In this case, the iGenda platform will optimize the work cycles of the institution, maximizing availability of Human workforce and other resources, resulting in advantages for the institution and the quality of the healthcare provided.

These scenarios require different types of tests and different types of implementations. The implementation will follow the typical test-improve method. In that sense, several personae were created for test purposes, each one with given roles, in a typical simulation platform. The personae were created with different demands, according to the specific purposes of each test. The validation was made by comparing the results of the system to the expected ones.

5.1 Results

The results of the implementation are depicting the failures and successes of the development path initially devised. The following examples represent a group of problems faced during development, the solutions adopted and the respective results. These solutions were tested in a simulation platform, with some students playing the several roles defined, in order to assess the behaviour of the whole system and cater for new developments. Thus, for the sake of realism, during the tests, each of these students represented one of the personas created. The use of the defined personas keeps the tests linear and sets a base pattern for the incoming results. This way, it was constructed a batch of possible and acceptable results to each persona, which were used to compare with the results of the simulation.

Two personas were created to modulate the typical users, a *young worker* and *aged person*. The personas were created with several options within the configuration of each one, following the most common characteristics of each target of demographics. For instance the *young worker* should have the FTM set up to the minimum possible execution. The results can be depicted as follows.

In the *young worker* persona the Free Time Manager was a challenge. To this persona, the free time should be totally controlled by him and the FTM should be a mere suggestive agent that should simply monitor the routines of the user and make suggestions in cases of free time.

In the *aged person* persona, results suggested that the family connection is not that important and the Free Time Manager was also a bit harsh in terms of scheduling. Moreover, the initial user interface was difficult to use by a person that was not a regular user of technology. The decisions of the Conflicts Manager in terms of rescheduling were also a bit offset and if another person was involved sometimes this person could not proceed to the event.

The Free Time Manager also showed a problem of spreading, i.e., if there are several short activities, e.g. if a user has 4 different activities of 30 min each on a single hour, this becomes more stressful than relaxing to the user.

Considering the Conflicts Manager, the reallocation of events did not always go as smoothly as expected. In multi-person activities, the rescheduling would not always occur as expected if another person involved had a calendar filled with activities.

Moreover, the notification of errors was not always as expected. In terms of interfaces, the development philosophy was to keep them simple and minimalist, reducing the interaction needed (e.g. buttons, options). In that sense, the entire configuration must be done by a technician. The quest for usability and adaptive interfaces continues and usability guidelines will be considered from now on. To highlight the main functionalities that the interfaces provide, sequences of screenshots of the outcome of several tasks are presented in Figs. 14, 15, 16, and 17.

6 Conclusions and Future Work

At this moment, this project follows several parallel lines of work. The main modules of the iGenda are fully developed and are already working in a beta state, allowing further higher-level services to be developed. Once the test phase is finished, an implementation in a real scenario is expected, using, at first, a selected controlled group of users. The rest of the modules will be gradually integrated as they enter a more mature stage of development, thus becoming available to its users. We expect CMS module to be the more challenging one to implement as it deals with medical real-life activities and, thus, risky environments.

Meanwhile, the strong acceptation of this project, by both the scientific and the medical community, encourages us to continue its development and proves that this is a valid path. Each new idea implemented opens new research doors and

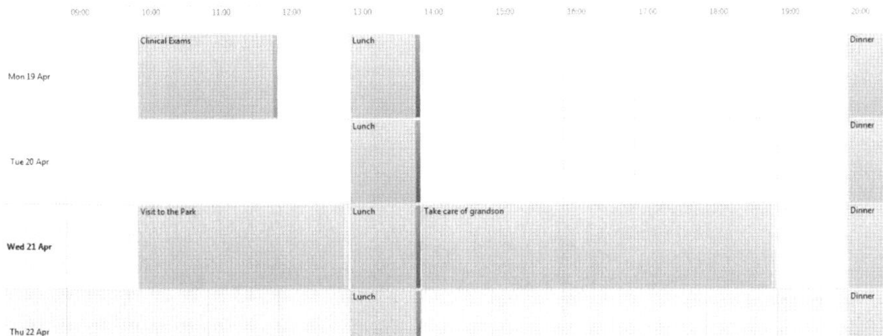

Fig. 14 Initial agenda with a few events

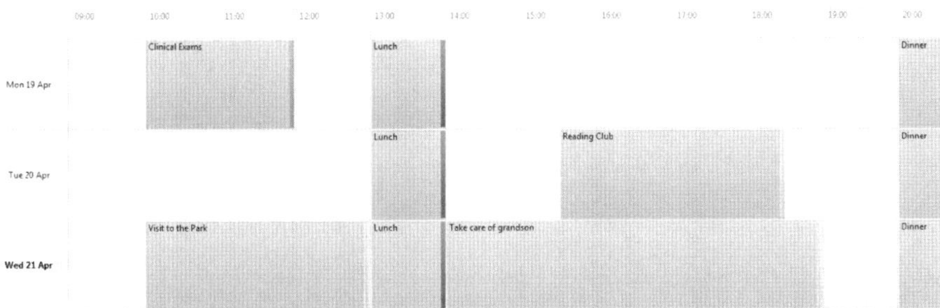

Fig. 15 Execution of the free time manager with a low spreading

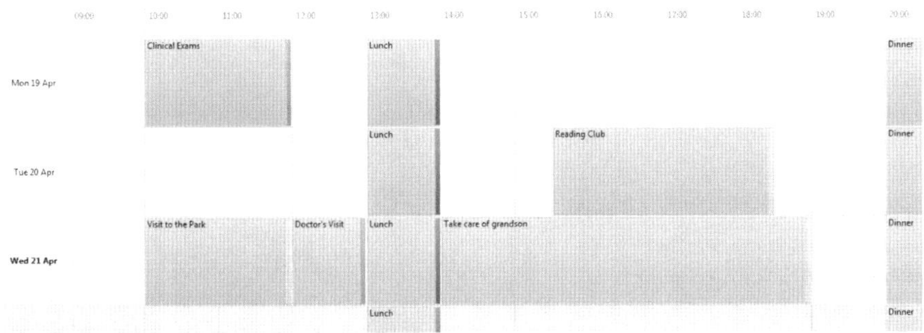

Fig. 16 A resizing of a non-important event with a scheduling of a priority 1 event

allows more functionalities, so possible future work is immense. Here, we include machine learning techniques to determine what combination or sequence of actions patients prefer. We are also considering the further development of the Sensing module in order to provide more information and possibly new ways of perceiving health-related problems and how to solve them.

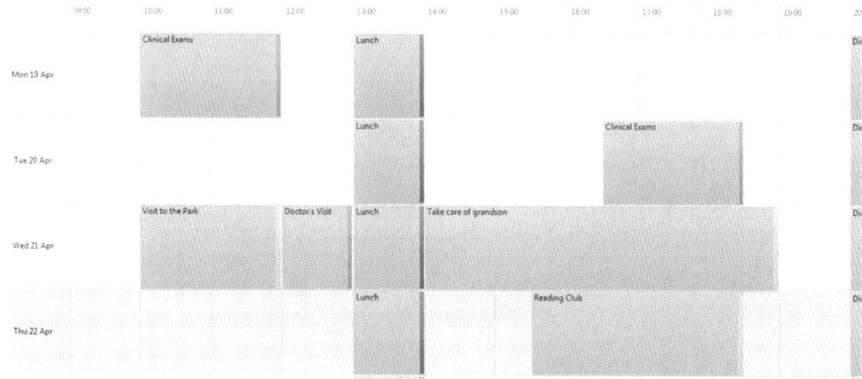

Fig. 17 Moving of a non-important activity and a scheduling of a priority 1 event

It is our opinion that the small common things that we do every day are the ones that really make a difference in our well-being. This project is a life changing one as the characteristics made available to the users are simple in its essence but of a great value, specifically when one considers patients with memory impairments.

References

1. UNFPA, State of World Population 2009, 2009.
2. Geda YE, et al. Prevalence of neuropsy-chiatric symptoms in mild cognitive impairment and normal cognitive aging: population-based study. Arch Gen Psychiatry. 2008;65:1193–8.
3. Charness N. Aging and human performance. Hum Factors: J Hum Factors Ergonom Soc. 2008;50:548–55.
4. Petersen RC, Negash S. Mild cognitive impairment: an overview. CNS Spectr. 2008;113(1):45–53.
5. Tucker G. Age-associated memory loss: prevalence and implications. J Watch Psychiatry. 1995,741–747 (Publisher: Massauchusetts Medical Society).
6. Addis DR, Wong AT, Schacter DL. Remembering the past and imagining the future: common and distinct neural substrates during event construction and elaboration. Neuropsychologia. 2007;45(7):1363–77.
7. Novais P, Costa R, Carneiro D, Neves J. Inter-organization cooperation for ambient assisted living. J Ambient Intell Smart Environ. 2010;2(2):179–95.
8. Ricardo C, Paulo N, Ñngelo C, José N. Memory support in Ambient assisted living. In: Luis C-M, Iraklis P, Hamideh A, editors. Leveraging knowledge for innovation in collaborative networks, vol. 307. Boston: Springer; 2009. p. 745–52. doi:10.1007/978-3-642-04568-4_75.
9. Jiang J, Geven A, Zhang S. Hermes: a fp7 funded project towards computer-aided memory management via intelligent computations. Berlin:Springer; 2009.
10. Hodges S. Sensccam: a retrospective memory aid. In: Proceedings 8th International conference on Ubicomp, 1 Edition Springer, 177–193 (2006)
11. Brown P. GC3: memory for life: getting things back. http://www.memoriesforlife.org/document.php?id=47 2004.
12. Ashri R, D'Inverno M, Luck MM. Agent-based software development. Norwood: Artech House Publishers; 2004.

13. Wooldridge M, Jennings NR. Intelligent agents: theory and practice. Knowl Eng Rev. 1995;10:115–52.
14. Moreno A, Valls A, Viejo A. Using JADE-LEAP to implement agents in mobile devices, Source:http://jade.tilab.com/papers/EXP/02Moreno.pdf. 2003.
15. Ball MJ, Lillis J. E-health: transforming the physician/patient relationship. Int J Med Inform. 2001;61:1–10.
16. Ñngelo C, Paulo N, Ricardo C, José M, José N. A memory assistant for the elderly. In: Papadopoulos G, Badica C, editors. Intelligent distributed computing III, vol. 237. Berlin: Springer; 2009. p. 209–214. doi:10.1007/978-3-642-03214-1_21.
17. Ñngelo C, Paulo N, Ricardo C, Corchado J, José N. Multi-agent personal memory assistant. In: Demazeau Y, et al., editors. Trends in practical applications of agents and multiagent systems, vol. 71. Berlin: Springer; 2010. p. 97–104. doi:10.1007/978-3-642-12433-4_12.
18. Fraile JA, Tapia DI, Rodriguez S, Corchado JM. Agents in home care: a case study. Hybrid artifical intelligence systems. Vol. 5572/2009 LNCS, Springer Berlin. 2009. doi:10.1007/978-3-642-02319-4_1
19. Teixeira A et al. Speech as the basic interface for assistive technology. In: DSAI'09, DSAI software development for enhancing accessibility and fighting info-exclusion, 2009.
20. Carneiro D, Novais P, Costa R, Gomes P, Neves J. EMon: embodied monitorization. Heidelberg: Springer; 2009. pp. 133–142.
21. Li K, Decker J. Coordinated hospital patient scheduling. In: ICMAS '98: Proceedings of the 3rd International Conference on Multi Agent Systems, 1998.
22. Syswerda G, Schedule optimization using genetic algorithms. In: Davis L, editor. Handbook of genetic algorithms. Van Nostrand Reinhold; 1991. p. 332–349
23. Dey AK, Kameas A, Ramos C. Thematic issue on contribution of artificial intelligence to ambient intelligence. J Ambient Intell Smart Environ. 2009;1(3).

About Motivated Project Teams, User Expectations, Proof-of-Concept Testing and the After-a-Good-Project-Hang-Over

Piet Verhoeve, Ann Ackaert, Jan Van Ooteghem, Jeroen Hoebeke, Maarten Steenhuyse, An Jacobs, Annelies Veys, Mieke Van Gils, Heidi Buysse, Stijn Agten, Brenda Aendekerk and Rina Vangerven

Abstract The sense of making good use of ICT applications in support of elderly care system seems all too obvious. However the actual adoption of such applications is very slow. It seems that good design, testing and intelligent value market analysis, are not sufficient to continue the life of many applications after the running-out of project subsidies. A Belgian multi-disciplinary team gained the hands-on-experience during two projects on this topic. This chapter describes these experiences and the lessons learned during the design, development and proof-of-concept testing phase in the field.

Keywords Homecare · Multi-disciplinary · Pilot · Field · Elderly · Video

P. Verhoeve
Televic N.V, Izegem, Belgium
e-mail: p.verhoeve@televic.com

A. Ackaert (✉) · J. Van Ooteghem · J. Hoebeke · M. Steenhuyse
IBBT–UGent/IBCN, Ghent (Gent), Belgium
e-mail: ann.ackaert@intec.ugent.be

A. Jacobs · A. Veys
IBBT–VUB/SMIT, Brussels, Belgium

M. Van Gils
IBBT–K.U.Leuven, Leuven, Belgium

H. Buysse
IBBT–UGent/MIG, Ghent (Gent), Belgium

S. Agten
IBBT–UHasselt/EDM, Hasselt, Belgium

B. Aendekerk · R. Vangerven
Wit Gele Kruis VZW, Limburg, Belgium

Commun Med Care Compunetics (2011) 3: 223–245
DOI: 10.1007/8754_2011_17
© Springer-Verlag Berlin Heidelberg 2011
Published Online: 14 June 2011

The sense of making good use of ICT applications in support of the activities of the daily live (ADL) of elderly people seems all too obvious. Meanwhile time adoption of these new services and applications in the healthcare market is slow, extremely slow in comparison with other sectors. Careful and user-centered design, proof-of concept testing and intelligent value market analysis, seem not to be sufficient to continue the life of many applications after running-out of project subsidies.

This chapter will describe the hands-on-experience and the lessons learned of a multi-disciplinary team in Belgium, who has elaborated from 2005 to 2009 two R&D projects in the field of eHomeCare services (respectively COPLINTHO [1] and TranseCare [2]). These projects involved research teams from different disciplines and with industrial and care organizations as project partners. The projects were co-funded by the care organizations, industrial partners and the Flemish IWT and IBBT subsidiary channels. Currently efforts are being made both by the involved companies and by the IBBT to bring some of the developed services to the market. How to cross this gap from projects to market is still a challenge in the eHomeCare area.

1 Description of the Project

In both cases the project consortium consisted of a multi disciplinary team of academic, non-profit and commercial organizations covering technical (academic and commercial), user (academic), legal (academic) and healthcare (non-profit) expertise domains. Both projects also aimed at putting co-development mechanisms into practice in order to enhance the co-operation between the industry sectors involved, the potential users, the non-technical and technical research groups. Each project was finalized by realizing a "proof-of-concept" demonstration during the second project year in order to illustrate in a live-environment the concepts developed for an innovative communication platform for the eHomeCare sector. The exact configuration and functionality of such a proof-of-concept demonstrator was each time defined by the end of the first project year.

The main objective of the COPLINTHO project was to study the introduction of ICT in the area of the home care (denoted as eHomeCare). Both technological and non-technological issues were taken into account in this project. The non-technical study covered a wide range of aspects such as regulation, liability, social impact and usability of the services (both for the caregiver as for the patient). The technical part of the project was devoted to research and development of several innovative ideas for the eHomeCare environment such as the creation of an ambient intelligent environment to support the care process of the patient, the creation of innovative communication platforms tailored to the needs of patients, nurses or homecare in general and the creation of secure and efficient data exchange services between all involved actors. In short, the COPLINTHO project aimed at bringing ICT to the homecare environment, more specifically oriented towards diabetes and multiple sclerosis patients.

The second project "TranseCare" narrowed down the scope towards people suffering from chronic diseases and/or from degenerative disabilities due to age. Although specific pathologies were encountered during the field tests (i.e. actual persons), the methodologies and concepts were developed based on the more generic categories such as chronic diseases and degenerative disabilities irrespectively of the age at which they occur. The objective of the TranseCare platform was to support these people through the aid of an ICT platform, focusing on real needs, and real life situations. The TranseCare project aimed at taking the concept of "independent living systems" a step further than mere R&D conceptual demonstrators. In short, the TranseCare project aimed at adapting the ICT towards the users instead of the other way round.

The project focused on three themes:

(i) The creation of a "transparent home environment", offering to users an "open window" on the world in their home environment through the aid of ICT

- An easy to reach "point of contact/central desk" supported with interactive video allows emergency or social calls (e.g. peer groups or communities)
- The study and development of game concepts integrated in this interactive video platform (occupational therapy, infotainment).
- Study and exploitation of the concept of virtual buddies. Stimulate social contact (with e.g. the "good morning-good evening service), decrease the feeling of isolation

(ii) The creation of a "transparent data exchange platform", offering the adequate information to both professional and family caregivers.

- The study and definition of data exchange flows for the required settings(medical, care)
- Semantic interoperability, both at the level of syntax or at the level of true information content
- Study and development of all necessary architectural components for the creation of a web-service based data exchange platform (privacy and security issues, authentication, authorization, advanced engines for dynamic workflow organization, development of a Patient Information Location Service)
- Study of all related legal and liability issues

(iii) The creation of a transparent network environment offering support to both domotica and mobility aspects

- Adaptation of Personal Network (PN) (self configuring and self organizing heterogeneous networks) concepts to the involved care settings.
- Use of proxy technology assessment techniques to collect and analyze user feedback.
- Research on PN-federation (the collaboration between PN's) to increase collaboration in between actors (e.g. patient and nurse).
- Study of all legal and privacy issues in this domain.

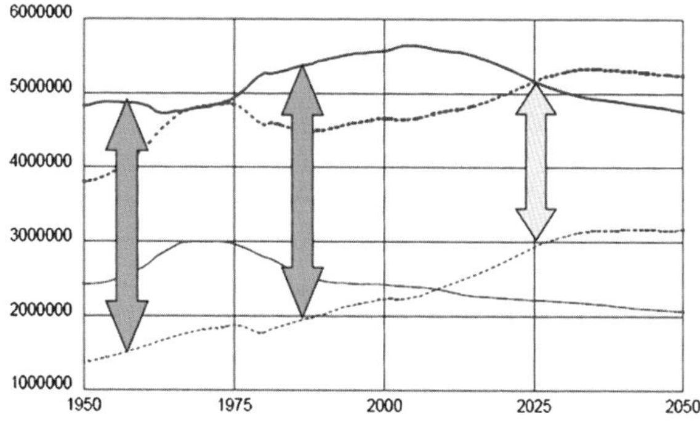

Fig. 1 Evolution of the population in Belgium (legend anno 1950:from top to bottom respectively age groups 20–59/dependent eldery an youngsters/ 0-19/60 +)

The result of both projects was a custom configurable eCare platform that connects to the users television through the Internet, and allows for video-telephony with a professional care help-desk, other users of the eCare system and informal caregivers using an instant messaging client on their PC.

2 Development of the Project

2.1 Arguments to Start the Projects

The major arguments for these projects were the societal challenges that have to be faced in the near future due to the ageing society. Indeed, already today there is a global shortage of qualified care staff, hospital and nursing beds which cannot only be solved by building more infrastructure or training additional persons in healthcare domains. Based on population numbers and predictions towards the future [3], the ratio of active persons compared to the care needing persons will drastically shift in the next decades; a ratio which has practically remained constant over the past century as indicated in Fig. 1. This figure shows the numbers for Belgium as an example, but they are applicable to each country in the western world. If the present model of care would continue, about half to two-thirds of the active population needs to be active in the healthcare sector by the year 2025.

While it is clear that not all elderly persons will be able to find a place in a nursing home, another societal change is taking place: both the elderly and society are more and more aware of the fact that most persons like to continue living at home continuing their independent lifestyle with specific care support provided at their location by professional nurse and family caregivers. Although this general user trend can be considered as a clear answer to the shortage in nursing homes, it aggravates the shortage of nurses since a home nurse also spends a lot of time traveling from one patient to another in case of homecare.

It should be clear that a change in the caring process will be part of the near future in order to be able to provide sufficient care for society. Although changing the care system is not part of the COPLINTHO nor of the TranseCare project which should be left to the healthcare professionals and governments, the multidisciplinary team was (and is) convinced that ICT can provide a supporting key role in making the healthcare process more efficient, providing more caring time for the nurses by reducing time spent on non-care activities and enabling communication process to exchange information electronically vs. paper based solutions. Examples of such efficiency enablers are:

- A better/faster communication between all actors involved in the care process; e.g. a home nurse stays up-to-date on the fact that a patient is admitted to the hospital so that she doesn't need to visit the patient at home, that the meals-on-wheels service is informed, etc.
- Video based communication that can be used to build a trusting relationship with a coordinating nurse without the need for that coordinating nurse to drive from home to home each time. In addition the video communication will give the nurse a better idea of the patient's condition compared to an audio only (phone) based scenario.
- Secure electronic communication between professional and non-professional caregivers.

2.2 What were the Goals/Expectations

As indicated in the previous section, the combined expectation of all partners was to gain a better insight and to advance the introduction of ICT technologies into the home care sector. This global expectation can be split into different more concrete goals, based on de different axes of the multidisciplinary team:

2.2.1 The Service Axis (Care and User)

The addition of telecommunication to the offered PAS-service [4] might possibly be of great value for the nurse/operator of the alarm central. With help of the camera, possibly by non-verbal communication, they are able to check on the patients room and make a better estimation of the patient situation. In this case the unnecessary call for help can be avoided (and vice versa).

The user expects a simple implementation with an ease to use and a flexible programming of the camera. Is this generation ready for this? When selecting the patients, we see motivated caregivers, however the user group (elderly) tends to reject the implementation of the technology (e.g. due to stigmatic effects), how can this introduction hurdle be circumvented?

Improving communication with the social networks of the users: not only on personal level (family and friends) but also care specific (medical staff, caregivers, coordination nurses, etc.)

2.2.2 The Technological Axis

The nurse and operator of the alarm central request a clear speak-listen connection, a good image quality, the possibility of the implementation of the patient file and the history of the calls. These items are needed to make a good estimation of the call which will be followed by the correct interventions.

Concerning our target group, we should be able to modify the program on request/demand since elderly users need specific, adapted offerings according to their needs in their specific condition which evolves over time.

Technologies should be based on open standards that the solution can make use of available networks such as internet connections and can integrate with existing systems in order to provide a smooth adoption path rather than requiring a big bang style conversion. In addition providing a system without explicitly creating a lock-in scenario is being preferred by most organizations (both profit and non-profit).

The projects aimed at implementing a data and information pull-technology based scenario from home care or hospital with specific access rights (social nurse, nurse, etc.) for all users. This had to be done by demonstrating actual electronic exchange of necessary data between hospital and home care in a secure and trustworthy style such that all users (both providers and consumers of information) will be inclined to use the systems.

2.2.3 The Business Axis

eHomeCare comprises a large number of actors, with not only different interests and motivations but also very different financial models (government, non-profit, commercial, personal relationship, etc.). Concerning the cost efficiency, video communication might serve as a filter at the alarm centres, thus providing a benefit for the care organization. However we can wonder if the telecom operators are ready concerning the financial part of lowering the costs of the connection fees and monthly rent.

Business modelling based on financial flows typically ends in very complex figures and dead end reasoning. Can a more simple framework be devised which will enable the introduction of ICT in home care environment.

2.3 What were the Innovative Elements?

The projects encompassed several innovative elements on the different axes of the multidisciplinary approach. They can be summarized as follows

2.3.1 Multidisciplinary Axis

As both projects encompassed a multidisciplinary team, the goals and expectations of each partner (stakeholder) were oriented in different directions. During the first project COPLINTHO, this proved to be a tedious process resulting in delays and complications to realize the demonstrator; the project even had to be extended in order to have a minimal field testing period. During the execution of the TranseCare project a specific "white book" methodology [5] has be devised based on the lessons learned during the COPLINTHO project. This approach not only allowed the different stakeholders to express their goals but also proved to be an efficient method that facilitated the discussions between technical and non-technical participants. Furthermore it enabled the projects to create a clear focus on the use cases, the user scenarios and the demonstrator from the early start of the project while allowing to adapt the specific conditions of the demonstrators according to the outcomes of the technological research tracks (which are by nature uncertain at the start of a research project). This "white book approach" consisted of first distilling specific user scenarios based on the goals and expectations of all partners, using the persona methodology [6–8]. Secondly the approach added a technological mapping to each scenario, which encompassed the relevant technological components and communication channels between the devices. In doing so, it was possible to estimate the technological risks of each user scenario according with respect to actually building the demonstrator. Furthermore this approach also allowed the non-technical partners to take an active role in the discussions as each technological setting was specifically linked to each user scenario. The result of this approach was that already in an early stage a clear consensus was created which classified the user scenarios and demonstrators to "field", "lab" or "concept" categories, thus managing the expectations of all partners, lowering the implementation risks in the field, and increasing the chances towards success at the end of the project.

2.3.2 Technological Axis

The communication platform studied en developed in the projects was not just about bringing the video communication to the end user, but it was about creating a solution that is fit for care. This means that the solution had to match a set of challenging requirements with respect to quality, safety, security, possibility^{TM} to install (by non-technical staff), usability (by non-tech-savvy elderly) and the legal framework (privacy and trust issues). During the sequential projects, the concept evolved from a healthcare terminal based design to the far less intrusive design of Xtramira^{TM} [9], which connects to the television set of the end user. The multidisciplinary research helped to create the innovative design of the user interface allowing for a practically manual free usage (by the elderly), while at the same time realizing a high trust factor concerning privacy issues ("can I be seen on the internet").

The Virtual Private Ad-Hoc Network (VPAN) [10] concept aims to securely and automatically interconnect distributed groups of devices. It aims to create secure self-organizing virtual networks in which any service can be deployed, shielded from the outside world. Since the services we want to provide involve different players (elderly, caregivers, family...), the interconnection of their devices in a user friendly and secure way is a key feature. Through this VPAN technology, multiple devices at distant locations that need easy access to each other's data and services are grouped in a logical, virtual, network. This is done automatically and securely, regardless of the heterogeneity of underlying networks. Based on security information, devices can verify if they are member of the same group, after which they can setup secure links to exchange information. The network will organize itself regardless of the location of devices and any movement of devices will trigger a reorganization without user interaction.

The technology also contains a service framework which automatically announces the availability of services to other members of the same group and allows user friendly access and management. Any network based service can be deployed on top of the logical network formed by the members of the group. As such, the VPAN technology effectively hides the technological complexity of the interconnection between devices and creates a permanent and closed group. Furthermore, the technology meets the flexibility requirements. Not only in terms of devices and services, but a device can also be member of multiple groups, which are all nicely shielded from each other.

The web based video enabled central desk can also be considered as a technological innovation. A new framework was developed that could realize a fully zero install (i.e. easier roll out conditions) application for the alarm centre central desk functionality. This application did not only implement audio and video but also realized a queuing/dispatching functionality for directing the alarm calls to the available staff. Additionally the application also encompassed a remote video camera activation toolset which complies to the legal requirement in the elderly homecare setting. Finally the application integrated a case management portal.

2.3.3 Care Axis

The innovation according to the care axis is the integration of telecommunication within the first line aid to develop supportive technology for caregivers, the nurse and other first line aid operators. This means that a better estimation of the problem can be made by telecommunication means. The technology created in these projects serves to guard the security of the user, taking into account the protection of the privacy of all users involved yet still allowing for efficient information exchanges to support the care process.

As was demonstrated by Arnaert [11], these projects also demonstrated that the use of video technology can increase the self esteem, lifestyle, well being and the participation of the patient to the society. In addition the results of both projects have indicated that this also applies for the family caregiver. Thanks to the ICT technology, more frequent (shorter) communications can be realized, hence providing a better understanding of the patient's condition and life, which results in a more comfortable feeling.

2.3.4 Business Axis

As indicated above, business modelling based on financial flows typically ends in very complex figures and dead end reasoning. The number of published value network models to evaluate the economic feasibility of eCare services is limited. A literature study and expert interviews have been executed. Studies on stakeholder readiness analysis [12] as well as a review of guidelines [13] and key indicators [14] for cost-benefit analysis [15] for telehomecare could be found, but are rare. During the projects, a multi-actor analysis indicates the benefits for all actors involved in the eCare ecosystem. The resulting mathematical model will help formulating a business case towards governmental agencies, insurance companies, healthcare providers or private investors as to how much and how soon to invest in eCare [16, 17].

3 Outcome of the Project

3.1 How and Why Did the Project Succeed/Fail

To measure the success of this we make a distinction between the experiences for the user groups and the experiences with the multidisciplinary project team and technology itself.

3.1.1 Multi Disciplinary Team

A success is definitely the cooperation and communication with the technology partners. Healthcare received a very good flow of information and support of the multidisciplinary team.

3.1.2 User Axis

In healthcare we need to make a distinction between 4 user groups: the elderly, his/her caregivers, nurses, and the operators of the alarm central since their expectations are different.

The operators of the alarm central were a little anxious at the start. They were fearing an increase of workload. A disappointing result was the patient enrolment for the TranseCare-study. For the test case of video surveillance only one patient met the enrolment criteria and gave consent. The inclusion criteria were very challenging and requested a single-living patient of the "Wit-Gele Kruis" organisation with a mobility score of 2 or more and a possibility of a toilet-visit score of 2 or more on the Katz and Weckx scale. A second reason for the low inclusion rate was due to the fear of the elderly for new technology. (see Sect. 6.1) The elderly person that was included, was very enthusiast at start. It should be remarked that we do not know whether this was due to the extra visits or due to the technology. She suffered from dementia, but had still good cognitive skills.

To search for test patients, one of the departments of the "Wit-Gele kruis" organisation was contacted. They were requested to "spread the word" and search between their patients for patients fulfilling the inclusion criteria. Although, at start they were very scared of the technology (see also Sect. 6.4), the nurse of the test person was very happy she tried out the technology; she gained confidence to use this type of applications. This is a success on a small scale since we first needed a convinced nurse before convincing the patient.

Although the caregivers of the test person were living at a short distance from their mother, they were very enthusiastic about the technology. They were excited to see their mother (in-law) on a screen and have more contact with her without the explicit need to frequently drop by in an unannounced style. The net result of this additional contact was that the caregiver was more at ease that everything was all right. Can we generalize this result? Can we conclude that this application is a success for the caregivers?

Although the technology components developed proved to be operational and successful, the dependence of eHomecare on external companies like for example the internet provider proved to created difficulties for testing. Not only the prices were not adapted, also when there was a connectivity issue it took too long before finding the problem (due to the many actors involved and the variability in modem install base) and solving it. Shortening problem solving times would make it easier to retain test persons. However when the users are asked whether they would like to adopt the technology, the price of the technology and accessories is very important [18].

From user point of view, we have the impression that the technology would be a bigger success and easier acceptable if it would be provided by packages (everything needed included); however even research based on prototypes, as in our cases, can provide valuable feedback for further and future product development. Another item to take into account is the fact that technology should be that simple that in case there is a small problem (connection issues etc.) the nurse can solve it.

3.1.3 Technological Axis

At the end of the COPLINTHO project, the terminal based demonstrator was at the same time successful and a failure. It was successfully designed, operational and proved to be an excellent demonstration that the multidisciplinary team could deliver actual results. Furthermore it proved to be a good "ambassador" into the market place, resulting in a steep climb of the reputation of Televic N.V. previously active in residential healthcare but not active and not known in the home care market. It was a failure due the fact that the user validation of the terminal proved to be not yet at the level of the end user skills (suffered from multiple sclerosis disease), and that it proved to be too stigmatic (having a healthcare terminal indicates that the user is dependent). Both aspects were considered as valuable lessons learnt for the second project TranseCare.

During the TranseCare project, the homecare vision was elaborated and a new concept was devised that focused on the non-intrusiveness and an elderly-proof usability without ending in stigmatic situation (neither towards the care dependency nor towards the especially-for-the-old label). This approach resulted in a device that combined the correct functionalities (social calling, alarming function and telemedicine) while being easy to use for the elderly and non-stigmatic at an achievable pricing rate for the target market (compared to existing non-video capable products). The device is currently commercially available under the name Xtramira^{TM}.

The VPAN concept successfully realized the whole set of specific requirements. It can be argued that they are or can also be solved by other existing protocols. However, these solutions only tackle one specific aspect, but fail to tackle the other requirements. Simply combining a number of these solutions is also too limiting in order to meet all requirements. This is exactly the strength of the VPAN concept, that it is an integrated solution that meets all requirements.

During the TranseCare project, the VPAN technology has been used to realize an end user scenario in a residential care setting at the "OCMW De Vijvers" organisation. The user scenario that was designed in close collaboration with the care providers (according to the principles of the participative design methodology [19, 20]) targeted the reinforcement of the communication between the elderly residents and the visitors (family and friends) by bringing the world outside the residence closer and cherishing the memories. By means of the VPAN technology a specific TV channel was added to the TV-set of the elderly person which allowed to exchange messages and pictures within the community of friends and family. The results of this experiment indicated that the application could indeed enhance a closer contact between visitors and elderly persons. Most elderly persons prefer many short contact moments compared with few long visits. The fact that the VPAN system allowed feedback (the fact that the pictures/messages had been seen) was considered a motivation to add additional content to the system, hence improving the contact. During the actual test period, this improvement was most prominent and satisfying for the users when connecting the elderly person with the grandchildren; this observation did differ from the initial assumption that it would mainly improve the communication between the elder and the oldest child (primary caregiver).

Although the both the application experiment at the "OCMW-De Vijvers" organisation and the VPAN technology proved to be successful, an actual go-to-market scenario has not yet been identified. The VPAN concept has also been used in other research projects such as Magnet and Deus.

3.1.4 Business Axis

During the TranseCare project we analyzed the economic viability of eCare solutions. A multi-actor analysis was executed, calculating for each actor, depending on the roles they are fulfilling, their costs and benefits in a dynamic way. A detailed analysis of all roles required to offer eHomeCare services was elaborated. Several business models have been analyzed and compared, where different provider take up a dominant role in delivering eHomeCare services towards the patients. The results show for the health care actors (general practitioners, home care and retirement homes) social benefits, either in terms of new customers, time savings or serving the needs of customers. The largest components of the tariff paid by the patients include call centre and network connectivity costs. The eCare infrastructure would ideally be subsidized by the government to enhance the speed-up of rollout of eHomeCare services. We concluded that all actors participating in the offering of the eHomeCare platform and services can benefit from the implementation of the system, which is of great importance to help formulating a business model towards governmental agencies, insurance companies, health care providers or private investors as to how much and how soon to invest in eCare.

3.2 Was the Project Continued?

As both projects were funded out of the Flemish research funds, which stops at proof-of-concept phase, neither project was continued as a whole. However, several aspects did continue after the termination of the projects:

The exchange hospital—home care is succeeded and the project will continue. Started from some "easy to implement" (but necessary) data to exchange, other data-exchange will follow. These phases however will proceed out of the context of a project. Because it is necessary, hospital and homecare will invest themselves.

The video communication device has been brought to the market as the "Xtramira™" and is actively being promoted by Televic Healthcare. At present the product has attracted the interest of the market, not only in the originally targeted homecare setting, but also in the residential elderly care market.

The video communication experiment has been taken up by a lead customer: OCMW-Kortrijk, which has evolved into a showcase on the living lab approach in Flanders [21]. Furthermore this experience has been taken to the European level in the context of the Apollon [22] project where the solution will be brought to the living lab in Helsinki, Finland.

The socio-economic modelling has received much attention from generic industry platforms on eHealth. There it will be investigated to what extend these results can be used in future scenario's to transfer terms as "better quality of care" into objective numbers which can be used for policy decisions.

4 Internal Influences on Development and Outcome

4.1 What Requirements were Expected from Those Involved in the Project

During both projects there has been a constant attention and continuous evolution with respect to the requirements. The white-book approach proved to be an essential tool to facilitate this process without ending up with projects where development is blocked due to constantly evolving requirements. During this process a number of "rules-of-thumb" were used as guidance:

- Focus on realistic goals: better less ambitious but possible than blue sky and nothing realized
- Don't forget the user requirements (compare to the technological); they need to be gathered for different elements within the communication network (alert system calls, multiplayer gaming, video chat application, …)
- Manage expectations across disciplines during the entire project cycle: what is expected from healthcare and what is healthcare expecting from its technological partners?

  More concrete the expectations in the projects can be summarize as follows:

- Healthcare is actively searching for technology working as an assistant of the nurse and/or as a facilitator for the elderly. As already mentioned the number of elderly is increasing faster that the number of nurses (see Sect. 2). Also, the elderly are more isolated in their homes since their social network is smaller. Hence the expectation of assistive technology. Healthcare expects a technology adapted to the user profile with an ease to use. Is the support of the technology matching the requirements of the user groups?
- The industry expects from the healthcare an actively participation with testing the applications, a constructive commenting and forwarding feedback concerning user experience and future expectation.
- The healthcare organizations are expected to actively search for test persons fulfilling the inclusion criteria and personnel.

4.2 How and Due to Which Causes Did Those Requirements Change During the Process

The very nature of both the COPLINTHO and the TranseCare project implied a change in requirements during the process. Indeed, since both projects had the combined ambition to advance user centred design of ICT services for home care as well as advancing the actual ICT technology at the same time, a conflict situation arises. This conflict can be illustrated by the fact that traditionally technical requirements are being drafted when user information is available while at the same time the user scenarios have to be created according to the possibilities of the technology envisaged. The mere fact that neither the technological development nor the user research was only finalized at the end of the projects implied a change in requirements.

Additionally the requirements are also influenced by the actual availability of test persons. Especially elderly homecare settings have to cope with difficulties due to ageing, increasing illness or worse. Based on the initial requirements, the healthcare organizations searched for test persons between their patients. However the enrolment criteria were very challenging. Is the user profile fitting the requirements of the application? Is this application suitable for elderly with dementia, or mentally impaired persons? Or everybody? Should the application be simplified? Do the users need a more simplified application?

The white book approach proved to be an excellent tool to manage this variability. It allowed to "softly" fix both user requirements and technological requirements at an early stage while providing sufficient room for adaptation as technological risks turned out to be not feasible or user selection to complex.

5 External Influences on Development and Outcome

5.1 Did Economic Aspects Play a Role in the Development and Outcome of Your Project?

As with any project, economics play a role in the development and outcome of the project. Both the COPLINTHO and the TranseCare projects had approved funding, however the funding level was different for academic, non-profit and profit sector partners (ranging from 100% to 0% funding). The fact that the funding mechanism was available proved to bootstrap this multidisciplinary project approach. Without it, there would have been little chance that such a diverse multidisciplinary team would be created in the Flemish context.

The economic aspects of the solution were explicitly taken into account during the projects. Not only the possible cost factor of the resulting solution but also the search for business models that can enable the eHomecare market to develop. Indeed, in the end the only economic aspect that is perceived by the end user is the price for that eHomecare user. We see that the elderly users of today are willing to use ICT-applications and that their acceptation is high. However, we should take into account that this is also only with a limited cost for these applications [23].

The search for a viable cost/benefit model for all actors involved to support and fund large eHomeCare projects will be crucial for the development of the Flemish market.

Fig. 2 Example of remote
control use by elderly:
typically two hands

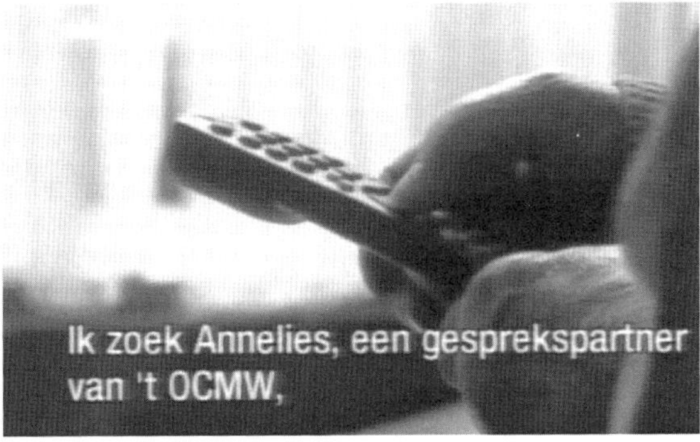

5.2 How Did the Project Development and Outcome Affect the Partners of the Project, Both Individually and as a Consortium?

The vision of industry and healthcare is traditionally opposite oriented; healthcare practices start typically from a user perspective with "watching" the patient; what are the patients needs; which type of technology is accessible (use and cost) for our target population? This is rarely the case for the ICT industry, which is typically oriented towards technology driven developments. Combined with the fact that ICT developers are typically young of age, the end result is often that product ideas are disconnected with actual situations and the target user group of elderly persons.

During this multidisciplinary collaboration a change in mind set was established on both sides

5.2.1 The ICT-Organisations Approached Care

By collaborating in the multidisciplinary team, the ICT organizations gained knowledge and better understanding of the actual environment and situation of the elderly persons. Examples can be found in the knowledge that retired persons are not very often confronted with new types of technology (hence have less adaptivity skills), that they have a different ICT-intuition and handling skills (e.g. hand–eye coordination for navigation or use of the remote control, as illustrated in Fig. 2) which gives the term "usable" a whole new dimension.

5.2.2 The Care Partners Approached the ICT Industry

By having to explain the needs and being involved in the development process, the healthcare organizations also gained knowledge and a better understanding of the industry driving forces. Examples of this process can be found in the increase in confidence that technology can be used when adapted to the user, the joined search for business models instead of the strict need to have cheap (free) technology for the end user.

The result can be summarized in the fact that the healthcare needs to gain confidence in the use of the technology and the application, the ICT organizations need to gain confidence in the fact that adapting to the (end) user environment can result into business and both sides need to gain confidence that the elderly can (and want to) participate and use the technology.

5.3 Did Legal Issues Affect the Development and Outcome of the Project?

Several legal issues were investigated during the projects, mainly focusing on privacy issues of all actors involved.

A first result of this study was to implement a specific feature in the video communication device (Xtramira^{TM}) that enabled the user to remain in full control of his privacy with respect to activating the local camera connected to the Xtramira device. In case of alarm condition, the local camera is automatically activated. A practice that fully conforms with legal conditions.

A second result of the legal study was that the field trial had to be limited to test with a system that only used a single camera for communication purposes. Hence, the scenario which encompassed multiple cameras that allow the desk caregiver to search for the elderly person by activating the cameras from a distance was demonstrated in realistic conditions but not actually used with end users during field trial.

5.4 Were Regional Aspects Involved in the Development and Outcome of the Project?

As the use of ICT does not imply strict regional limitations to the deployment of the eHomecare service, regionality was not taken into account for the field trials in the COPLINTHO project. Although this demonstrated the possibility to roll out ICT based eHomecare services over a large territory, it should be considered that healthcare always has a local/regional component that needs to be taken into account. Indeed, providing physical home care implies a regional organization, hence the current a regional structuring of care coordination.

During the TranseCare project, a more regional approach was taken, which not only proved to be more close to existing care structures but also proved to be more practical to cope with technical field trial issues.

If ICT is to be successful in the home care domain, it has to respect that existing organizational structure, i.e. supporting the home care rather than implying a new organizational model. When ICT will prove to support and enable additional efficiencies, the care organizations will gradually and automatically adapt their structures to a larger regional scale.

6 User Aspects

6.1 Did (possible) Implementation of Your Project Involve Educational Challenges? If So, How were They (to be) Met?

A first educational challenge was met during the early stages of the projects. Indeed the multidisciplinary team combined members with very different backgrounds and all were confronted with specific terminology: not only the traditionally difficult technological terms and acronyms but equally confronting were the specific healthcare terms and scales. A nice example of this conflict in terms can be found in the term "protocol"; used in a technological context it designates a method by which different devices communicate; in the healthcare context it is being used to designate specific steps in a treatment or care process. Each time new members were added to the multidisciplinary team, specific time had to be spent in order to close the gap and reach a sufficient level of understanding.

Educational challenges were also encountered at the level of the test persons (both elderly and nurses): research has shown that the current group of elderly is willing to accept or adopt new technology if this is improving their quality of life. However, what they do not want, is to lose control of their choices (freedom) or their privacy. The TranseCare project involved a camera, internet (i.e. equipment that was introduced into the home by the project) and the use of their own television (already present).

The educational challenges encountered by the healthcare organization were specifically related to the approach to enrol test persons into the project. The enrolment procedure used had to be adapted such that it did put more emphasis on the unchanging privacy and the personal freedom of the test person to accept or decline a call. The need to learn more about the technology behind the application itself was not present, so this was not extensively explained.

A first contact to enrol a patient was by phone. During this phone call we checked the interest towards the project. We noticed a lot of "scared" persons that seemed to have reservations towards the use of technology, which could be caused by the mental state of the person contacted. However, the initial phone call starting with the message "This is the alarm central speaking..." was too invasive and confusing for the person being called. To keep the link between the alarm central and the project, it was decided to call the primary caregivers instead and ask whether his/her parent/family member/neighbour could be interested. If the primary caregiver gave a positive indication, the question was asked to contact the elderly person and to discuss the basics of the project. If interest remained, a personal contact between the elderly person and healthcare was organised. This change in approach was vital to convince possible test persons to join the test program.

For future cases, it might be useful to search for test patients by contacting the leading nurses of different departments instead of only contacting one as was the case in the projects. The holistic approach to care by the homecare nurse is often sufficient to get an estimate on the capabilities and/or interest of the patient.

We also noticed that it usually were the children of the contacted person that were enthusiast about the technology and were trying to convince their family member.

Another, long term, educational change should be made to the training of the nurses. At present, most nurses are confronted with this type of technology for the first time during their actual working situation. It should be more efficient to inform them earlier, e.g. during their school education period. The sooner they realize what technology can bring to them, their patients and his/her environment, the easier it will be to convince them to try the technology themselves and to support their patients.

6.2 Were User Satisfaction and Usability Part of the Project's Goal and How?

In eHomecare user satisfaction is an important means to gain the confidence of the users. As mentioned before, research has shown that the "upcoming" baby boomers are very interested in technology. However, the research also concluded that these potential users want to use technology if their freedom and privacy is guaranteed. The current elderly population (prior to the baby boomers, also called the pre-war generation) has grown up with little or no technology adherence and with a "natural" fear for this technology. Therefore this pre-war group needs especially the product satisfaction to gain confidence.

Hence, both user satisfaction and usability were part of the projects from the start, however the focus was more oriented toward user centric design and evaluation by user rather than big statistical user satisfaction studies. For each demonstrator that was build, specific attention was given during the design and development process to realize a solution that could meet the user expectations and could also be used by the non-tech-savvy end users. Already early in the development process user feedback was achieved based on low fidelity prototypes (mock ups, paper printouts of the screens, etc.). The usability of the first operational high fidelity prototypes was evaluated during a lab test under controlled conditions with test users in observation rooms. During the field trials, a similar user evaluation was executed; however extensive observations are less obvious in the field. Hence the feedback was triggered using in depth interviewing techniques in order to get insight in the user motivation.

The result of this approach was a successful evaluation of an easy to use central desk application as well as the easy to use interface of the Xtramira^{TM} device. Actual observation tests with different test persons with ages ranging from 57 to 75 clearly showed that 90% of the test persons could execute the test sequences based on the embedded instructions, without any additional training.

Fig. 3 Creative user
methods to safeguard privacy

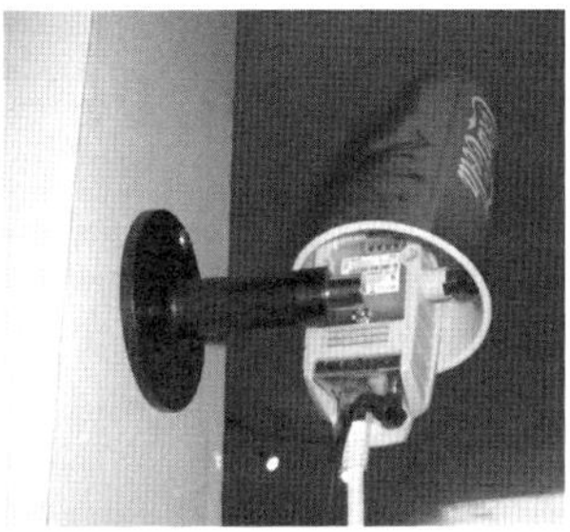

6.3 Did User Aspects Influence the Final Outcome of the Project?

During both projects user aspects were constantly balanced with technological requirements in order to create the multidisciplinary solutions which the projects targeted. In order to gain insight in some specific user aspects, field observations were organized to study comparable products to create a funded understanding of the user context. More specifically a study of the knowledge of the symbols used on the buttons of phones and remote controls was performed in order to provide recommendations for the development of the Xtramira^{TM} symbolic language and remote control.

As both projects also used cameras at the user's premises, specific attention was given to study the reactions of the test persons with respect to this feature. The research showed that especially the presence of the camera was disturbing, resulting in strange attempts to safeguard their privacy by covering the camera, as shown in Fig. 3. The fear of having someone to see their homes trough the camera when they do not know and losing control is for the contacted persons too high to accept/adopt the technology. Therefore, the final design of the Xtramira^{TM} was adapted to include a very small camera in order to easy the user in getting used to the system without being constantly focused on the large lens in the living room. Additionally the application interface of the Xtramira^{TM} was modified in such way that it is obvious and intuitively clear to the end user when the image is being transmitted to the other side.

6.4 What were the Reactions from Users on Your Project?

To fulfil the inclusion criteria, the test user had to be a patient of the "Wit-Gele Kruis" organisation in the Limburg-province, he/she should have on the Katz-Weckx scale a mobility score of 2 or more, toilet visit of 2 or more and should live alone. These criteria are not easy in that way that most of these patients have troubles with using the technology themselves. When contacting the caregivers to check for their interest, the most common comments were "this is nothing for my parent. He/she is too scared and too confused to use this application." "It will disturb her/him too much." "She/he is not using the phone, this will be way too difficult for her/him". One patient that fulfilled the enrolment criteria gave informed consent to participate to this project. She and her family were very enthusiast to use this application. After installing the application at her home and solving the first technical challenges, it became clear that she was too nervous to use the system. It was difficult for her to understand how to accept or start a call. The mental state of the user worsened faster than expected. The system was removed when it was too disturbing and confusing with respect to the mental state of the test person.

To find patients, a call and visit were made to a department of the "Wit-Gele kruis"-organisation. The leading nurse checked the general patient list and discussed with the nurses of that department on her weekly meetings the requirements. Every nurse checked between his/her patients to see whether there was a patient fulfilling the criteria. On general, these nurses reacted very positive on the new technology although they were very scared as well to use the application. They were scared to "break" the system and that the help-line would not be enough to solve an issue when it would occur. Some of them even "hoped" that they would not have a patient, so they did not have to manage the technology. The nurse of the actual test person was also worried, but very enthusiastic as well. She managed very well to start the application, comfort the patient and help her to sort her mind when the test user was disturbed. The nurse mentioned also that the sound should be easier adjustable for the hearing impaired.

For the alarm central, that receives all calls of the personal alarm system, it was not difficult to use the system, but still too disturbing since the alarm was used together with the usual alarm system. Using both systems next to each other could cause an overload of work.

The test users with respect to the social contact scenarios were very positive as the solution was perceived as a decrease of the social isolation. This effect was observed at the side of the elderly person but also at the side of the children and grandchildren. In one specific case, the use of the system even realized the granddaughter to get interested into details of the earlier life experiences of her grandparent, an aspect which was unknown and had not been addressed earlier by the granddaughter.

Most test users were also very positive with the non-stigmatic combination of social contact communication and alarming device that was enabled by the Xtramira^{TM} solution.

7 General Aspects

7.1 Did Your Project Have an Effect on Matters Like Efficiency, Quality of Labour, Quality of Care and Quality of Life?

Neither the COPLINTHO project nor the TranseCare project had specific tasks during the project to objectively evaluate matters such as efficiency, quality of labour, care and life. However, based on the results of the field trials and the positive responses of the different users, positive effects are to be expected. In case the project results would be deployed on full scale, they would certainly increase the quality of labour for the central desk nurses at the alarm central organization. The same result is expected for the caregivers as the system allows for a more personalized touch and the time gain due to video communication will normally be converted into additional time spent with the patient. During the project a family caregiver mentioned a similar effect, i.e. spending more time on the actual communication rather that a very short visit due to travel times.

As the video system also allows for a better understanding and insight in the patients situation and environment, it is easier to quickly grasp the seriousness level of an alarm (or the lack of in case of false alarms). This results in a lower dispatching rate in case of false alarm, hence resulting in a better use of the care staff.

As indicated before, the increase in social contacts and the breaching of the sense of social isolation (made possible through the solutions created in the projects) resulted in a sense of better quality of life for the users.

7.2 *What Kind of Dissemination Strategy Did You Develop/Use?*

During the project, several dissemination strategies were used. Besides the traditional publications along the multidisciplinary domains, specific workshops and seminars were organized. The purpose of these events was twofold: dissemination of the results and creating awareness in the homecare sector, as well as using the audience as sparring partner to get feedback on the approach taken. This effect was most prominently present in the workshops relating to the business modelling.

Additionally a portable version of the demonstration set up was also shown at several local care events, hence creating the awareness that technology can provide a benefit to the homecare sector.

Finally a short movie was made at the end of both the COPLINTHO and the TranseCare project. Each time the movie tells the story from the viewpoint of the end user (i.e. patient, nurse, family) and demonstrates how the solution and technology can support the healthcare process.

Although creating such a movie was a tedious task and involved skills not present in the project consortium, the reactions of the different audiences proved that it is very effective in communicating the results of multidisciplinary projects which tend to be complex to explain. It even proved to be an effective marketing tool during the early market introduction days of the Xtramira^{TM} product.

8 Conclusion

The results of the multidisciplinary projects COPLINTHO and TranseCare clearly illustrate that this approach can be very successful to create solutions that bridge the gap between the high tech world and the homecare world. The methods developed and used during the projects prove that it is indeed possible for tech-savvy and non-tech team members to learn to understand each other and to collaborate in order to design solutions adapted to the end users.

Although there are still hurdles to take in order to fully bring the resulting solutions up to a full scale deployment, the results clearly illustrate that technology in homecare belongs to the near future. These solutions give opportunities for the elderly at home to broaden their social network; in a time where families become smaller, and people become more individualistic, video communication opens a window to the world and can provide access to a higher quality of life.

Acknowlegment The results presented in this chapter were based on the successful collaboration of the COPLINTHO and TranseCare partners: IBBT-UGent/IBCN, IBBT-UGent/MIG-RAMIT, IBBT-V.U.B./SMIT, IBBT-K.U.Leuven/CUO, IBBT-K.U.Leuven/ICRI, IBBT-UHasselt/EDM, Wit-Gele kruis VZW, Televic N.V., Medibridge N.V., Custodix N.V., Androme N.V., AZ-St. Elizabeth, UZ Gent, In-Ham VZW., Solidariteit voor het Gezin VZW.; both projects were partially funded by IBBT and IWT.

References

1. COPLNTHO acronym stands for: innovative communication platforms for interactive eHomeCare.
2. TranseCare acronym stands for Transparant ICT platforms for eCare.
3. Centraal scenario van de vooruitzichten 1995–2050, Nationaal instituut voor de statistiek, Federaal Planbureau, 1996.
4. PAS: personal alarm service, an existing service that allows the user to activate an alarm and set up a phone communication with a central desk nurse which can dispatch help if needed.
5. Yogesan K, Bos L, Brett P, Gibbons MC, editors. Handbook of digital homecare, a multi-disciplinary approach towards the design and developmen ot value$^+$ eHomeCare services. Berlin: Springer; 2009.
6. Cooper A. The inmates are runing the asylum. Indianapolis: SAMS; 1999.
7. Caroll JM. Making use: scenario-based design of human-computer interactions. Cambridge: MIT press; 2000.
8. John P, Tamara A. The persona lifecycle: keeping people in mind throughout product design. San Francisco: Morgan Kaufmann; 2006.
9. www.xtramira.com.
10. Hoebeke J. Adaptive ad hoc routing and its application to virtual private ad hoc networks, Ph.D., ISBN 978-90-8578-172-1, NUR 986, Ghent: Ghent University, 2007.
11. Arnaert A. Tele-nursing for the elderly, the case of videotelephone care, explorative study, Ph.D. Leuven: K.U.Leuven; 2001.
12. Hebert MA, Korabek B. Stakeholder readiness for telehomecare: implications for implementation. Telemedicine J e-Health 2004;10(1):85–92.
13. Dávalos ME, French MT, Burdick AE, Simmons SC. Economic evaluation of telemedicine: review of the literature and research guidelines for benefit–cost analysis. Telemed J e-Health 2009;15:933–948.
14. Rojas SV, Gagnon M-P. A systematic review of the key indicators for assessing telehomecare cost-effectiveness. Telemed J e-Health 2008;10:896-904.
15. Dansky KH, Palmer L, Shea D, Bowles KH. Cost analysis of telehomecare. Telemedi J e-Health 2001;3:225–232.

16. Van Ooteghem J. Multi-actor analysis for identifying the economic viability of eCare solutions, to be presented at medicine 2.0 conference, November 29–30, 2010, Maastricht, The Netherlands.
17. Van Ooteghem J, Ackaert A, Verbrugge S, Colle D, Pickavet M, Demeester P. Economic viability of eCare solutions, to be published in the proceedings of eHealth 2010 conference, December 13–15, 2010, Casablanca, Morocco.
18. Onderzoek uitgevoerd door het Centrum voor Publieksonderzoek van de KU Leuven, in opdracht van het Vlaams Instituut voor Wetenschappelijk en Technologisch Aspectenonderzoek (viWTA): Kleurrijk vlaanderen kleurt grijs, eindrapport, Leuven, juli 2004.
19. Bijker WE. The social construction of technological systems; new directions in the sociology and history of technology. Cambridge: MIT Press; 1987.
20. Sleeswijk Visser F, Stappers PJ, Van der Lugt R, Sanders EB-N. Contextmapping: experiences from practice. CoDesign: Int J CoCreation Design Arts 2005;1(2):1–30.
21. NEXTlab project, funded by IWT (2010–2012).
22. Apollon, FP7 project, www-apollon-pilot.eu (2009–2011).
23. Telecare voor ouderen: socio-economische analyse van het gebruik van video-telefonie binnen de ouderenzorg/Peetermans Annick, Hedebouw Georges, Pacolet Jozef, Devoldere Paul, D'Haene Filip, Pouillie Roland, et al. Leuven: Hogeschool instituut voor de arbeid; 2004.